Birth Wisdom

Tricks of the Trade
Volume III

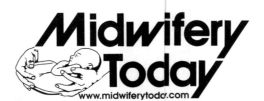

Birth Wisdom
Tricks of the Trade, Vol. 3
by Midwifery Today, Inc.

Disclaimer: The content of this publication represents the opinions and practices of individual midwives from around the world. The practices are not researched, approved or endorsed by Midwifery Today, Inc., and its staff members. Before employing any methods you may wish to use, confer with your peers, know what the current medical practice is in your area, and study the available research for risks and benefits. And of course, consider the specific client circumstances, using your own professional judgment as to the appropriateness of any given method. The editors and publisher disclaim any liability arising, whether directly or indirectly, from the use of this publication.

Published by Midwifery Today, Inc.
P. O. Box 2672
Eugene, OR 97402 USA
(541) 344-7438 / In U.S. and Canada (800) 743-0974 / Fax (541) 344-1422
E-mail: inquiries@midwiferytoday.com   Web Site: http://www.midwiferytoday.com

Editor-in-chief: Jan Tritten
Cover photographs: Tia Browder
Layout design: Elise Kimmons
Cover design and design editing: Jennifer Rosenberg
Managing editor: Bobbie Willis
Layout design assistant: Ken Ackermann
Copy editor: Nancy Olson

All rights reserved. No part of this book may be reproduced or transmitted in any form or by any means, electronic or mechanical, including photocopying, recording or by any information storage and retrieval system without written permission from the author/publisher except for the inclusion of brief quotations in a review.

Copyright ©2001
by Midwifery Today, Inc.

Library of Congress Cataloging-in-Publication Data
Midwifery Today
    Birth Wisdom: Tricks of the Trade, Vol. 3

    ISBN 1-890446-06-8
    I.   Title
    1.   Midwifery – United States
    2.   Childbirth – Pregnancy

This book is dedicated to all the midwives, doulas and childbirth educators who openly share their experiences and insights with others that we all may be better birth practitioners. If you have a trick to share, send it to Midwifery Today.

Toward Better Birth

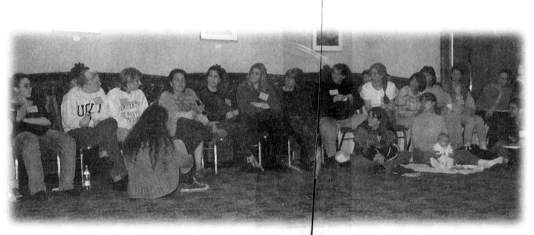

Tricks of the Trade circle at the Eugene 2001 Midwifery Today Conference

Contents

Philosophy of Care
- Trust Builds a Shelter 7
- The Spoken Word 8
- Walking a Fine Line 9
- Integrating Waterbirth Into Maternity Care: An Agent for Change 10
- Building a Successful Midwifery Practice 12
- Transport Etiquette 13

Remedies
- The Amazing Alfalfa 15
- Herbs for Use in Pregnancy, Birth and Postpartum 16
- Herbs for Emotional States 17
- Heartburn Treatment Alternatives 18
- Homeopathy: What It Is and How to Apply It 19
- Black Cohosh: Uterine Effects 21
- Bottoms and Births 22
- Urinary Tract Infections 23
- Herbal Allies for Childbirth 24
- Traditional Chinese Medicines for Hemorrhage 26
- Chinese Patent Remedies for Hemorrhage 30
- Homeopathic Remedies and the Midwife 32
- Grieving and Healing: Miscarriage 33
- A Holistic Approach to "Loose Cervix" 34
- Herbal Protocol for Group B Strep 36

Prenatal
- Teaching Moms About Prenatal Nutrition 37
- What Can Midwives Do? 39
- The Dance of Childbirth 39
- Land Food, Sea Food, Brain Food 40
- Holistically Meeting the Challenge of Infection 43
- Calendars, Clocks and Choices 45
- Relaxation for Pregnancy and Labor 46
- Postdates vs. Postmaturity: An Overview 48
- Emotional Factors in Prolonged Pregnancy 52

Labor
- Important Things I've Learned About Birth and Midwifery 53
- Prolonged Labor: Past and Present 55

Preventing Prolonged Labor 57
Twins: A Very Special Occurrence 62
A Study Outline on Twin Pregnancy, Labor and Delivery 64
Natural Alternatives to Induction 67
Sterile Water Blocks for Back Pain in Labor 72
Birth Balls 73

Birth
Normalizing the Breech Delivery 75

Immediate Postpartum
How Long Is Too long? 81
Hemorrhoid Prevention and Treatment 82
Controlled Cord Traction 82
Postpartum Bleeding 83
Can We Really Use Super Glue Instead of Suture? 84
The Vitamin K Question 86

Newborn Care & Breastfeeding
Kangaroo Care: Why Does It Work? 89
Cuddle Up! Slings and Baby Carriers 90
Milk Angels 93
Breast Yeast 95

Artists, Authors and Photographers

Suzanne Arms	Gail Hart	Holly Richardson
Cindy Belew	Chris Hafner-Eaton	Jennifer Rosenberg
Mary Bove	Judith Halek	Barbara Noble Schelling
Tom Brewer	Valerie El Halta	Maryl Smith
Caroline E. Brown	Valerie Hobbs	Anne E. Stohrer
Jill Cohen	Betty Idarius	Paula Tipton-Healy
Abigail Connelly	Joy Johnston	Jan Tritten
Kathryn Cox	Sharon Glass Jonquil	Nancy Wainer
Sabrina Cuddy	Marnie Ko	Gert Welsh
Rahima Baldwin Dancy	Sue LaLeike	Cynthia Yula
Judy Edmunds	Anna Lipo	
Anne Frye	Linda McHale	Special thanks to
Roberta Gehrke	Kiki Metzler	Sundance Natural Foods
Lisa Goldstein	Michel Odent	and Down to Earth Home Garden
Barbara Harper	Patti Ramos	& Gift

All uncredited photos by Jennifer Rosenberg and Elise Kimmons.

From the Editors

Jan Tritten, Publisher/Editor-in Chief

"Tricks of the Trade" is a favorite feature of both Midwifery Today's magazine and its conferences. All of our magazines and conferences include these tricks of the trade. I know each of you has many tips of your own that you can share with others, and we hope you will look into your practice and send us your own tricks and ideas.

This is a rich sharing of birth practice, and this sharing is brought to you in the third volume of our *Tricks of the Trade* series with the greatest hope and prayer that the birthing experiences of others will help you in your holy work of serving families.

My personal interest in this type of sharing came very early in my midwifery practice. I was an apprentice midwife attending my 17th birth. I was with another apprentice who had been to only 25 births. Our senior midwife had just found out that her ex-husband, the father of her child, had been murdered, and the birthing mom was pushing when our senior midwife called to tell us that she couldn't come to the birth.

My colleague was catching the baby because she was a little more experienced than I, and she was also a nurse. Baby Sarah's head came out, sucked back against the perineum, turned purple and failed to restitute. Yes, you got it—classic shoulder dystocia.

My friend could not get the baby out. I had just read in another magazine a trick by Ina May Gaskin that Ina May had learned in Guatemala.

"Monika, turn over to your hands and knees," I said.

My strong, German, soon-to-be midwife partner turned onto her hands and knees, and out came Sarah, who 23 years later is now my friend.

I don't know if anything in these pages will provide you with an answer to something as dramatic as this. In fact, I hope you never have to face something like this. I do hope, though, that in your constant efforts to know more and to be better birth practitioners you will find many ideas to help you improve your practice.

LOVE jan

Jan Tritten

Jill Cohen, Associate Editor

One of the best parts of midwifery are the many tricks you develop over the years. Each birth gives you new insights and ways. It is in light of this that Midwifery Today has presented its *Tricks of the Trade* series.

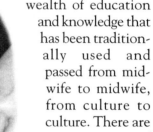
photo by Patti Ramos

We have collected, over many years, hundreds of tricks that midwives from all over the world have used. These tricks are the core of midwifery. They represent a wealth of education and knowledge that has been traditionally used and passed from midwife to midwife, from culture to culture. There are so many aspects of pregnancy and birth. And of course, there is a trick for everything!

My hope would be that you use this book wisely—applying well the tricks presented in this volume, just as they are well applied by those who share them here, knowing that each person is an individual and that one trick will not apply to all.

I have personally tried many things offered in this book and have found some great aids. I hope that from this reading you will enjoy, learn, be provoked to think and experience the thrill of a good trick at work. I also hope this book will inspire you to acknowledge your own potential to create and modify tricks to help the women you attend. Be sure to write and tell us of those tricks so that we can keep the tradition of *Tricks of the Trade* going.

Toward better birth,
Jill

Jill Cohen

Philosophy of Care

Trust Builds a Shelter

by Jan Tritten

TO TRUST BIRTH, midwives must first have a good, solid, thoughtful practice as their foundation. As Sister Angela Murdaugh says, "Don't practice 'wish midwifery.'"

We all know unexpected things happen in birth, ranging from difficult to devastating, but fearing or avoiding them should not be the substructure of our practices. Knowledge, practice, understanding intuition, practicality, and especially love are the foundation blocks; trust is the shelter built on that solid foundation. With the practitioner's skills assisting her, a mother can best prepare for birth by building trust in her body and herself, trust in her midwife and family, trust in the birth process, and trust in her baby. Trust shelters the mother from fear that something is wrong, from hurry and disrespect, from unnecessary interventions, and from fear of her own weaknesses or shortcomings.

I have been fascinated by the outcomes some of my colleagues have in their practices. Valerie El Halta, Judy Edmunds and Mabel Dzata, for example, all have very few transfers from home or birth centers to hospitals, and their outcomes for mortality and morbidity are also superior. They are not sacrificing mother or baby in order to get their impressive stats. Each of these women has a deep and abiding trust in birth, women and God. They work intensely with their women throughout pregnancy and during birth, trust is established and problems are taken care of. They all believe love makes babies come out, and without a doubt, each radiates deep and genuine love.

Mabel has been working in a hospital for more than three years now and gets the same outcomes she did when she was a homebirth midwife. Even though the birthing women she works with are strangers at first, they have fast labors and successful births. Mabel uses the same kind of respect and sense of privacy for the woman and her family in

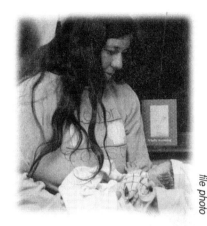
file photo

the hospital that she maintained at homebirths. In her eyes, respect is paramount to all human relationships and is the most important element in the birth relationship. Without it, trust can't develop, first between midwife and mother, and then in the process of birth itself. She does little things to maintain calm and respect, like keeping the door to the room closed and knocking when entering. She asks the woman's permission before doing routine procedures. By her own calm demeanor, she calms the hospital staff. Soon everyone is trusting that this birth will be normal. You don't have to get on the hospital treadmill of panic behavior or certainty that nothing will happen without intervention.

Good midwifery knowledge and skills on the part of the midwife and a woman's trust in her midwife's skills are other important aspects of her care. As Valerie says, "You must recognize and correct the 'orange warning lights' or you will have full-blown problems. Situations turn into problems and problems into emergencies." If a pregnant woman is developing early signs of preeclampsia, the midwife needs to know what she is eating and work with her on her diet to increase her protein and salt intake. There is no need to panic, no need to do anything but use your skills wisely and trust the woman's process. In the case of symptoms of early labor, keep a cool head and take the proper steps: analyze her diet, her stress level and her life. Help her toward health before a successful birth outcome is jeopardized. Is the baby posterior in labor? Try Valerie's technique to turn the posterior before the head is jammed into the pelvis (see *Midwifery Today*, Issue No. 36). Mind the orange warning lights and trust birth—not necessarily the textbooks, many of which need to be rewritten.

The road to wisdom means you will suffer much and surrender more, but you will witness many miracles. Trusting in birth is the best shelter to offer your pregnant and birthing women, and the best tool you can pull out of your birth kit.

Tips & Tricks

Language
The language you choose is important. Touch is important, too, but first ask the woman if she is comfortable with it. At the first exam, tell the woman, "Everything is going so well—your body is perfect!" Use positive language and constant encouragement. Be absolutely real with her.
Tricks of the Trade Circle, FL '97

Organizing & Educating
Develop slide presentations of birth photographs and create a powerful and informative presentation to give at schools, public events and conferences. This is a very effective way to inform your community about midwifery and natural birth.
Jan Tritten & Jill Cohen

Respect
Respect the mother and her pregnancy and birthing experience. Let her know she is Queen of the Day. Find ways to protect her from intervention and disrespect.
Tricks of the Trade Circle, FL '97

Be Personal
Call women by their names—it shows warmth and most people respond to it very positively. It seems so simple, but we often forget to do so.
Tricks of the Trade Circle, FL '97

The Spoken Word

by Linda McHale, CPM, and Barbara Noble Schelling, CPM

Empowering women to birth naturally is the midwife's most important job. One of the most powerful tools we can use to get the job done is the spoken word.

What we say to the pregnant women we attend helps them shape their birth experience. Positive affirmations and an upbeat attitude help make the impending birth joyous and achievable.

Unfortunately for most pregnant women, we live in a society that is addicted to drama. The mainstream media continue to help satisfy the addiction with their sensational stories about birth. Pregnant women, especially sensitive to worrymongering, are all too often regaled with horror stories, rumors and unverified "facts." A woman's mother warns that she will bleed too much after birth—so she does. Her sisters tell her she needs an epidural—so during the birth she turns to drugs because she believes she needs them. Birth that goes well is not as dramatic as the one that ends in cesarean or the marathon labor followed by the drug that saved the day.

Suppose that a pregnant woman's friends and caregivers tell her she can and will birth the way she needs to. Suppose we tell her she can birth without drugs, dependent only on herself and the love and support of her family, friends and midwives. If we prescribe wellness, strength and wisdom, she will be well, strong and wise! When we tell women that they know how to birth, they believe it because it is true.

From the very beginning of our relationship with a pregnant woman, we express our confidence that pregnancy and birth are not an illness but in fact a joyous occasion. At the first prenatal we encourage the couple or woman to ask all the questions about bad outcomes they can think of. We then tell them what we would do to handle each situation—how we would react; procedure and causes for transport; what equipment, drugs or herbs we would use; and if we have ever dealt with this situation before. Unveiling scary events helps allay fear. Sharing true stories about other women/couples who have faced these experiences puts them into a manageable perspective. We also tell the client that no one can promise them a perfect birth and baby. We will do our job as best we can, but in reality, some things are out of our hands. Once fears have been exposed and addressed, the client can feel free to put them behind her.

During the remainder of a woman's prenatals, we concentrate on positive birth stories. These true stories are powerful affirmations. We especially like to describe the humorous and touching moments we've experienced at births. "The baby always comes out" is the underlying message of these stories.

Noticing and exclaiming over signs of good health and fetal growth give the mom confidence. We praise her weight gain, beautiful skin and shiny hair, and the proud way she carries herself and her unborn baby. We see it and we say it. We support her efforts to educate herself by reading and watching birth videos, and talk with her about what she's learned or answer any questions she might have. Something as seemingly simple as the use of a bulb syringe is worthy of a few minutes of discussion. When she sees that she can make a choice about such a procedure, she feels confident and in control. This kind of verbal interaction done ahead of time frees her to be able to surrender during the birth.

A woman's previous births deserve plenty of discussion. If we attended these births, we can build on the positive relationship we had earlier on. No matter how many times a woman has given birth, there is always something she would like to do differently. Hearing herself talk about new ideas reaffirms her sense of self-empowerment. If previous births were satisfying, our job is easier because there is nothing like a good birth experience to bring on another. If a previous birth did not go so well, she has the opportunity to talk out what she felt happened to interfere with the process. Coming to terms with a particularly difficult birth is an ongoing process and will take time and plenty of feedback. Careful and respectful listening is essential.

Reminding the woman that every birth is different allows her to start anew.

Near the end of a woman's pregnancy, we invite all the women due around the same time to get together. Everyone enjoys the camaraderie, and no one is pressured to talk. Experienced moms tell their birth stories. "Yes, I give birth," she is saying. First-time moms hear good birth stories and in return pass on the special wonder and anticipation that is theirs. As each of the women in this group births, we tell the others as we see them at prenatals.

This is, of course, a time to be careful and discreet with your words. Sometimes just a birth announcement is enough; there's no need to mention the long labor, cesarean or congenital defect. Details can be learned when they meet again postpartum.

During birth, the words you say are even more important. It's essential to be careful not to prescribe the kind of labor we feel is best. It's good to be supportive, but not to make it conditional. Remind the woman that she is "doing it," that she knows how to birth. Affirm that she is handling it well.

If she is having a hard time, acknowledge it; remind her to do only one contraction at a time. Describe a hard contraction as a "good" one. When you make suggestions, tell her why the shower feels so good, why a walk will move things around, why a change of scene is good, why you're going to give her some privacy, why making deep sounds will open her up. Use positive statements to get affirmative actions; avoid "don'ts."

Some of the strongest statements at a birth are not words, but sounds.

Breathing together, whispering nurturing noises mothers make to their children are powerful utterances of love and support. And the very fact that we are there with them, holding them and nodding our heads as if to say "yes, everything is as it should be" is the supreme positive affirmation.

At birth, we love to hear affirmations from the baby. We hardly ever use our Dopplers prenatally, but we have found that at the birth the sound of baby's heartbeat is calming and reassuring. The baby is a very active participant, and we frequently speak directly to him or her: "Mommy loves you and wants to see you; it's OK to come out now." After the birth we thank the baby for doing such a great job.

Midwives can help mothers birth, but only the mother can deliver the baby.

Giving her sincere praise, respect and admiration is totally appropriate. She needs to be told that she has done something wonderful and that she is a good mom.

> **Doula Opportunities**
> Work as a doula in unwed mothers' homes, where there are high numbers of abused women.
> *Tricks of the Trade Circle, FL '97*
>
> **Soften Your Hands**
> Old Japanese midwives were said to have very soft, young-looking hands because they handled placentas, which are good for skin health.
> *The Japanese Midwives, FL '97*

Sister midwives, we must remember how powerful words can be. If we truly believe in the power of birth, it will be reflected in our speech. Remember to have a happy birth-day!

Walking a Fine Line
by Nancy Wainer, CPM

AT A RECENT hospital labor support, the laboring mom had a persistent cervical rim. Because she had expressed an interest in homeopathics during one of our pre-labor visits, I pulled out my bag of remedies just as the obstetrician walked in. "What is it that you have there?" he asked. I explained that it was gelsemium and told him that in many circumstances it quickly, safely and easily melted rims. He asked me several other questions and then said, "I have heard about homeopathy but I know very little about it. It would be great to find something besides Pitocin that helps dilation." He talked with the couple, and with his consent we used the remedy. Within a few moments the rim had disappeared and the mom was pushing her baby into the world. Later I chatted with the doctor and he asked if I would be willing to compile a bibliography that would help acquaint him with homeopathy for pregnancy and delivery. He shook my hand and told me it had been a pleasure working with me.

Three days later I was at the same hospital with another laboring couple. They were using a different obstetric practice, and their primary OB, who was agreeable to homeopathy, was not the doctor on call. When the obstetrician walked in and saw my bag of remedies he went ballistic. "What do you have there?" he yelled. "What right do you have to bring medicine into this hospital? Who has given you the authority to give drugs to this woman?" When I began to respond he shouted, "I have never even heard of such things and I don't want to know about your bag of tricks. We do not use those voodoo things around here." When the laboring mom said that her OB—his partner—had agreed to the use of remedies, he said, "Well I'm not her and she's not here." Thoroughly miffed and equally disgusted, he ordered Pitocin and an epidural and arrogantly strode out of the room.

What I do to offer labor support is influenced by how strong/insistent the mom is at the time and who is the doctor on call, as well as other factors. I have been at some hospital births where I have been encouraged to do perineal support and deliver the baby's head. One doctor handed me a pair of scissors to perform an episiotomy. I said, "Thank you, but I don't need them—I don't use them." He was astounded. He later told me that in 14 years of practice he has never NOT done an episiotomy. At other births in the same hospital I have not been allowed to do perineal support or be anywhere near the woman's vagina. One doctor told me to be more liberal with the olive oil I had brought, and another told me that if I opened the container he would have me kicked out of the room.

The biggest discrepancy in policies seems to be about turning posterior heads. I have been encouraged to not only "work Val's magic" (see *Midwifery Today*, Issue No. 36, "Posterior Labor: A Pain in the Back," by Valerie El Halta) but to please instruct the staff how to do it! At other times I have been told it is illegal for me to touch the woman, even with her permission.

I do not go into hospitals to argue, wage war or do battle. I tell all my couples what I am capable of doing in most circumstances and what may be beyond me—or simply not permitted—in a hospital setting. I ask them to discuss detailed matters of the birth with their OBs, warning the couple that if that particular doctor is not on call every one of the agreements may be rescinded. Sometimes I have a skill or a remedy or suggestion that might make a tremendous positive difference at their births, but I am not at liberty to do/use it because of "hospital policy." I have to remember that the couple chose the hospital setting for the "safety" and "comfort" it provides, and that they are then subject to the rules, regulations, boundaries and limitations that that choice means.

I know I make a difference. I do as much as I can to help make each birth as sacred, loving, gentle, peaceful, empowering, connecting and celebratory as possible. With the threat of Nubain, Pitocin, epidurals, cesareans and egos looming so closely, it is not necessarily an easy thing, but it is the best I can do.

Integrating Waterbirth Into Maternity Care: An Agent for Change

by Barbara Harper, Midwife

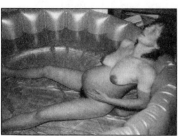

photo by Patti Ramos

A GROWING CONCERN expressed by many practitioners and birth activists is that consumers just aren't taking the lead in asking for the changes necessary to bring about safe and gentle birthing practices. But while this may be true in some areas, it is not true when it comes to waterbirth in clinical settings. The waterbirth movement has largely been motivated by women's requests for the comfort and relaxation that water-assisted labor affords.

Those services that are now offered in scores of hospitals across the Unites States have been accomplished without the cooperation and collaboration of nurse-midwives, nurse managers, physicians or administrators. In the past three years I have helped more than 60 hospitals—all with active nurse-midwifery practices—to establish waterbirth services.

Waterbirth reflects a philosophy of birth rather than a modality or a way of giving birth. Waterbirth is woman centered. Birthing in water was a woman's invention, even if men claim to have "offered" it to women. It was the women who refused to get out of the bath at the time of birth. I have heard many midwives reassure their clients that if their labor has progressed well and the mother chooses to stay in the water at the time of birth, the midwife will be there to support them in their choice of birthing in water, even if the midwife has not previously attended a waterbirth. The major factor assisting midwives in making the decision to support their clients in this choice is the increasing availability of educational materials, conferences and retrospective data on birth in water. The majority of published data on waterbirth is coming from England, where in April 1995, more than 1,100 midwives, nurses and physicians gathered to share their experiences of waterbirth from around the world.

During the last decade, in a push to make birth appear more "family-centered," tubs were installed in newly remodeled LDRPs (labor, delivery, recovery, postpartum), though there were major design flaws. They are usually too small, too narrow, and in too small of a space to allow women to experience the natural comfort that water affords. Nurses have been reluctant to offer women a bath because of the problems associated with getting a woman out of bed, off the monitor, undressed and into the water, only to discover that she is not really comfortable there. There have also been unnecessary restrictions placed on women with ruptured membranes, even though a 1959 article titled "Does Bath Water Enter the Vagina?" and published in the *American Journal of Obstetrics and Gynecology* states quite plainly that the practice of restricting women from the bath during the later days of pregnancy, and especially in labor, is unwarranted. Another concern for hospital personnel has been the possible transmittal of HIV and hepatitis. There have been several published studies, including statements from the Centers for Disease Control, concluding that the likelihood of transmittal in water is non-existent.

Allow me to illustrate how the process of integrating waterbirth into hospitals has taken place in two different locations. Lynn Springer is the perinatal coordinator of a small maternity unit at St. Elizabeth Community Hospital in Red Bluff, California. She was introduced to waterbirth by the nurse-midwife who is in practice there. Lynn immediately took hold of the idea of offering water to her laboring patients, but was blocked by the logistics of installing permanent tubs and not having enough room. She consulted architects, went to plumbing stores, picked out the jacuzzi tub and then set about to remodel a room in which to place it. In the meantime she arranged for an in-service for the nursing staff and a separate in-service for the medical staff taught by a physician who was actively offering waterbirth at his birth center. She consulted with her insurance providers, infection control department, materials management and the OB committee. In consulting with my office to arrange the nursing in-service she told me, "This is the easiest way to let women know they have some control over the [birthing] process....I will do anything to not only get a tub into my unit, but to start to offer waterbirths. I don't care how long it takes me." Her determination paid off.

One of the first waterbirths that took place was transforming for the whole staff. A young teen mother came to the unit

(Continued on next page)

Livestock Tanks

Many of the families in my practice area have not been satisfied with the shallowness of a regular bathtub for waterbirthing. I now use a livestock tank—it is Rubbermaid plastic, quite light for its size and deep enough so that an adult sitting in it can be submerged to her neck if she wants to be. It can be easily transported in the back of a Jeep, truck or van. In exchange for its use, I ask the birthing family to be responsible for scrubbing and bleaching it before and after its use.

One person approached a farm store that sells the tanks and asked to rent one. When the manager found out she was going to use it for birth, he let her borrow it free of charge. Give it a try!

Roberta Gehrke, MT

and was extremely fearful. At one point in her labor she was found hiding under the bed, but as soon as she got into the water she was able to calm down, relax and let go of her baby. Lynn watched as this frightened child became empowered and blossomed into a mother, noting that it never could have happened outside of the tub with such ease and dignity for the woman. It took close to two years to accomplish the feat of getting all 15 physicians who practice there ready to assist with waterbirth, but today everyone on the staff has done at least one waterbirth and the statistics indicate excellent outcomes in the 150 waterbirths that have happened to date.

Jade Kaplan, a CNM at Harris Regional Hospital in Sylva, North Carolina, gave a wonderful presentation at the Greensboro, North Carolina, waterbirth conference in April 1996 on the problems encountered in establishing a waterbirth study in this rural Appalachian facility. Jade had attended a number of waterbirths in her homebirth practice prior to joining a physician in his hospital-based practice. She knew the efficacy of water and had a request from one of her clients for a waterbirth in the hospital. The waterbirth took place without problems until the rest of the nursing staff, especially the nurse manager, discovered the fact.

She complained that there was no protocol in place in order to meet hospital accreditation standards. Because this is frequently given as an obstacle for starting a waterbirth practice, I have written standard protocols that can be adapted to any practice. These sample protocols were adapted by Jade's hospital, sent to nursing for approval, but rejected on several occasions. At the same time the OB committee approved them in the original form, but then rejected the revised set. In Jade's presentation at the conference she illustrated her talk with a diagram that indicated the circuitous route and the length of time it took to "officially" offer waterbirth. The project was finally accepted on the condition that only 10 women would use it and then the outcomes would be evaluated. After 20 water-assisted births in a portable pool, the hospital has now installed a permanent tub. The main requirement that got the program under way was providing an in-service for the entire staff. Education is the key to instituting any change in standard hospital practice.

Because the entire staff of these two hospitals was involved in the process, the nurses and administrators were introduced to the broad subject of gentle birth and woman-centered care. That is part of the magic of waterbirth in hospitals. The pool itself creates a protected environment that keeps technology at a minimum. Staff members who witness a waterbirth report that they find it difficult to justify the use of epidurals, pain meds and monitors when they know how beautifully and easily water works. Dianne Woelke, a nurse-midwife in San Diego, reported that the epidural rate dropped dramatically when they created a protocol stating that a woman must be offered a bath before getting an epidural. Once the women get into the bath, if it is big enough to move around in, they seldom want to leave, and soon forget about requesting an epidural.

Water-assisted labor is making an impact on birthing practices in hospitals and is providing a platform for addressing change. We watched midwives in England go through a scare in 1993 when the Royal College of Obstetricians and Gynecologists tried to stop waterbirth by publicizing that babies were dying as a result of the practice. The negative publicity only sparked more interest and made the world waterbirth movement more cohesive, directly leading to the first international symposium. Waterbirth is now taking place in hospitals in 37 countries that we know of. When waterbirth is accepted, it implies that women have a blanket acceptance and the ability to birth independent of assistance and technology.

Many practitioners find it hard to accept waterbirth for this reason. The rationales for using so much technology don't seem to "hold water" after witnessing beautiful births in water where all the physician does is take the photographs.

Tips & Tricks

A Baby in Every Classroom

Have a plastic pelvis and a plastic baby that negotiates this pelvis in every public and private school in the United States. It should be equipment as basic as foursquare balls. Start with one unit of teaching and rotate it through every classroom each year. Inspired teachers may want to purchase their own model for a year-round sensory display. Once it is purchased, the instigating midwife or parent should recheck every year to make sure the model has been in all classrooms.

Can you imagine what a terrific psychological impact this could have on so many young minds? Children can grow up pushing that baby through the bones, and it will become ingrained in their consciousness that the baby fits!

Linda Lieberman, OR

Strengthen Your Hands

One day the Midwifery Today staff were chatting about how midwives need to have strong hands to perform midwifery maneuvers with ease. Here's a few suggestions for strengthening hands and fingers: play piano scales, type, knead bread, unscrew stubborn jar lids, squeeze lemonade by hand, give your friends deep massages, pull weeds, sew by hand, thumb wrestle, learn pottery-making.

Jill Cohen, Jennifer Rosenberg, OR

Political Action Strategies

Get a bumper sticker that supports midwifery. I'm surprised how many people ask me what a midwife is. My bumper sticker has also led to my getting new clients and to speaking engagements.

Jill Cohen, Jan Tritten, OR

For more waterbirth information, contact: Waterbirth International, P. O. Box 1400, Wilsonville, OR 97070. Phone: 503-682-3600; Web site: www.geocities.com/hotsprings/2840;

E-mail: waterbirth@aol.com.
Waterbirth stories:
www.well.com/user/karil/Frame.html

Building a Successful Midwifery Practice

by Paula Tipton-Healy, LM, CPM

My midwifery path began more than 20 years ago, while working toward my bachelor's degree in nutrition. As part of my degree, I was to do a nutritional study of a particular group in society. Choosing to work with pregnant women, I found a general practitioner doing homebirths who allowed me to work with his clients. Through my connection with him and his practice, I started attending births, soon realizing this was my calling.

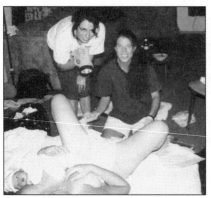

photo provided by Jill Cohen

After training with him, I then worked with a midwife in Colorado, and within a few years I was practicing on my own. If someone had asked me during that time how I would start and run a midwifery practice, I'm sure I would have drawn a complete blank. My thoughts were fully centered on being the best midwife possible and enjoying the unfolding miracle of birth. This privilege was so intense that I felt I would do anything and everything to be a part of it. The majority of years training to be a midwife are concentrated on honing our skills, nurturing our intuition and birthing ourselves as caregivers. The art of running a business with financial stability, success and professional integrity comes much later, along with wisdom and experience.

Many years ago, after being in practice for some time, I woke up one morning and realized the importance of being paid appropriately for my midwifery services. This was a shift in consciousness regarding how I viewed and valued myself and midwifery, which from the beginning has always been for me a labor of love. That day I came to realize my own self-worth and financial worth as a care provider. Once I made that shift in my self-perception, I was amazed to see that the families I served followed suit. As I began to place financial value on my skills, experience, education and services, my clients did as well. My acceptance and ability to receive their gift of payment created an even deeper sense of satisfaction from the births. What a gift this has been for my clients, as well as my family. (Of course, I have always offered a sliding scale fee for those less fortunate and have done a certain number of pro-bono births each year.) I relate the financial health of my practice to the counseling I give to moms: we must take care of ourselves in order to take care of others.

As midwifery teachers, we can integrate this understanding of value exchange into our apprentices' training by teaching them to understand their own self-worth as midwives. Learning to value their services and skills from the onset of their education will be an invaluable asset to them as they start out in their own midwifery practices. I strive to do this in several ways:

1. Pay apprentices—they provide a valuable service to me and to my clients.
2. Treat them respectfully, both in private and while with clients.
3. Have them assist in the financial aspects of the business. In my practice my apprentice is responsible for the collection of payments.

Most midwifery practices develop through a process of natural evolution. You may start out as a doula or childbirth educator and may spend time doing a midwifery apprenticeship—all of which will contribute to making a name and reputation for yourself—before evolving into a practicing midwife. As you begin to birth your midwifery practice, I recommend taking the time to clearly visualize yourself in a successful midwifery practice. Picture your practice in as much detail as possible. Next, spend some time writing down your goals. How many clients do you intend to serve in a year? How do you plan to present yourself and your practice? Is there a special client base you wish to target? Taking the time to clarify your plan will help you immensely as you begin to make choices for developing your practice.

Remember as you start to build up your practice that it is important not to take on more than you can handle. It can be very tempting as a beginning midwife to want to serve every woman who crosses your doorstep. But to be successful and provide quality care to your clients, you need to know your limits, and remember that it's OK to say no.

In addition to writing out the specifics of your business plan, it would be a great idea to make an affirmation collage for yourself. Draw or assemble some pictures that fit your image of your midwifery practice, and add several positive statements to yourself about the direction and success of your future practice. You can be as creative and expressive with this collage as you wish, and the affirmations should be inspirational to you. When you have finished the collage, place it someplace where you will see it every day to remind yourself of your positive vision for the future.

When you are ready to start making choices about your practice, one of the first issues you will need to address is creating a space. Your work space should reflect your style of practice and the level of personal connection and professionalism that you want to project. Many midwives choose to practice out of their homes. Should you decide to practice from home, it is a good idea to have some degree of separation between your home life and your business practice. For instance, your family should understand that when you are seeing clients in your home you are at work, and they should not interrupt you during appointments if at all possible. This will help you to present yourself as a professional and will allow your clients to feel that they have your complete attention during their scheduled appointment times.

(Continued on next page)

You may want to designate a room or other portion of your house as your office, to further enhance the professionalism of your practice. An alternative to working from home would be to rent an office space, either on your own or in conjunction with other midwives or health care practitioners. Regardless of where your work space is located, you should be sure that it is convenient for your clients to travel to for appointments, and that there is ample parking for them so they don't have to walk long distances to reach you. Also, if you are renting a commercial office space, be sure that it is in a safe neighborhood where your clients and their vehicles will not be at risk.

Once you have a space, the next step is to create an attitude for your practice. This attitude should be reflected in your appearance, manner, surroundings and how you conduct your practice. It is important for building a successful practice that your clients feel they are treated respectfully, that they have confidence in you and your practice, and that they feel safe in your presence and in your space. However, these goals can be accomplished in many ways; every midwife is unique, and your practice should reflect who you are as an individual. Midwifery is such a personalized field, it is essential that your practice and your work space are consistent with your personal style and values. If you try to fit yourself into a mold that is incongruent with who you are, your clients will notice the discrepancy, and the perception of it may negatively affect their ability to trust you.

Your clients will be your most valuable asset in terms of building your practice, so it is important to maintain good relationships with them throughout their care and afterward. Some good suggestions for providing continued support to your clients after their babies are born are to offer well-woman and well-baby care, acknowledge birthdays, and coordinate picnics and support groups for moms. I would also suggest that you work to keep up good relationships with clients who leave your practice for some reason; they may not continue in your care, but they may still refer others to you. In addition to all of this, it is also imperative to advertise if you want to expand your client base. I strongly recommend placing an ad for your practice in your local Yellow Pages.

Many women, upon learning that they are pregnant, immediately turn to the telephone book to locate midwives in their area. A Yellow Pages ad will also provide a reliable back-up source for your telephone number and for any other advertising you may choose to do. If you can work it into your budget, invest in running ads in local newspapers or periodicals. Plan your ads so that they reach the most people in the community you want to target. If you are trying to target a specific clientele, find out whether they have any localized publications in which you could advertise.

Even more effective than printed advertisements in building a practice is to make public relations appearances in the community. Volunteer your time to speak about midwifery and homebirth at childbirth classes, churches, La Leche League meetings, and local high schools and colleges. You might even put together a slide show or film to supplement your talks. Such appearances will help to raise the community awareness about birth options, and people will become familiar with you as a local professional. Most people feel more comfortable going to someone for care if they have had a personal experience or encounter with that person, or if someone they know and trust has personally interacted with them. You would also do well to contact your local health food stores, and spend some time talking to the managers of the vitamin departments. People often ask for referrals at their health food store, and a personal contact there could go a long way to building your practice.

Finally, I would recommend fostering professional relationships and referrals with obstetricians, perinatalogists, pediatricians, family practitioners, general practitioners and midwives, as well as building professional contacts and relationships with the other allied health professionals in your area. By this I mean chiropractors, acupuncturists, massage therapists, osteopaths, homeopaths, herbalists and health clinics. Many women who choose homebirth will also seek care in these different modalities. Your clients will appreciate your ability to give referrals to other health care practitioners, who in turn will refer their clients to you. Your practice history and reputation, advertisements, public appearances, and professional relationships are your keys to creating a presence in your community, through which you will build a successful midwifery practice.

Editor's Note: *This article is reprinted by permission of the author from the* California Association of Midwives News, Summer 1998.

Transport Etiquette
by Anne E. Stohrer, MD

IT IS USEFUL for direct-entry midwives to have an idea of what we "on the inside" of the medical system expect at transport. Sometimes the policies, procedures and mindsets are impossible to understand, but often with time and effort the process of transports can be made easier.

The primary ingredient for a successful transport is communication. I believe open and honest communication best exists within a relationship that is established and ongoing between midwife, client and physician. In my case, the direct-entry midwives in my area sought me out for a cup of tea. This informal meeting turned into a question and answer session on "What would you do if...?"

When I agreed to provide backup for them, our first transport was a client whose outcome was good, but whose labor course and cesarean were as frightening to me as to

(Continued on next page)

the attending physician. The midwives and I did not talk together, I became angry, and after the birth I sent them a furious letter concerning control issues. The midwives' immediate response was to invite me to join them for another cup of tea to talk about what had happened and how we could do better, and to acknowledge my issues about the birth. That conversation opened the door to my own personal growth regarding client/transport issues and paved the way for assisting with other births.

Important Visit

The second component of communication involves a pre-birth visit with the client and her partner. I use this time to try to establish rapport with the client, because an open relationship cannot begin in the middle of labor or after a transport. At our meeting, I ask about important birth issues, allow time for questions to be raised, and give them a handout about the policies and procedures at our hospital. I also encourage a visit with a staff pediatrician, a tour of the birthing center, and pre-registration, to head off middle-of-the-night client/partner separations for paperwork.

An added feature of these visits is that they allow both the client and me to decide whether or not we will be able to work together should a transport occur. Based on our pre-birth visit, I have refused backup to several clients for various reasons, including hostility or adversarial behavior.

Give a Call

Whenever a transport is considered, a call to the backup physician is in order. This gives the doctor the opportunity to arrange her personal life (I have three small children, for example), review the client's chart, notify the birthing center staff and prepare mentally. The early call also allows the midwife and the backup physician to talk over issues that may be impacting the labor, or to plan strategies to prevent the transport.

Making a Decision

The decision to transport is usually made by the client, her family, the midwife and the physician. It is always better to transport too early rather than too late, erring on the side of caution. Of course, my corollary is that it is always better to transport during daylight hours rather than at 2 a.m., when everyone has run out of energy and ideas. Often, we can predict transports hours before they actually happen. In my case, because I have to deal with pediatricians who do not support my homebirth practice, it is easier to explain 36 hours of ruptured membranes rather than 72 hours.

It is also easier for me, as the backup physician, if the client is prepared emotionally and psychologically before and during the transport. The midwives for whom I provide backup talk in a positive manner about me, the birthing center, and the decision long before the client arrives at our door. As midwife Ina May Gaskin says, go in presuming good will, and often good will results. If the decision to transport is truly made by consensus, then reinforcing that idea helps make transport easier. The client's arrival is a time for first impressions. Sometimes, the nurses in our birthing center are supportive, sometimes they are not. It is extremely important to understand that these nurses work within a technological center. Often, their sense of what is safe and right comes from different sources, such as hospital protocols. This is when the use of language becomes paramount. Phrases such as "If it is possible…" or "We would really like…" or "We have a pre-agreed upon birthing plan with our physician" work far better than an adversarial approach. When all else fails, fall back upon the idea that these people want a good outcome, too; they are just in a different place.

At our birthing center, a 20-minute fetal monitor strip is mandatory, but then if all is well, the belts come off and intermittent auscultation is used. All centers have their own rules and protocols that are absolute and those that are "bendable." It is the midwife's task to differentiate between the two in her backup facility.

I also explain to the client once again that it may take up to two hours for her to "own" the place where she is. I call it a "cool down" period, and speak of "cocooning" into a place where she can birth. Not all places acknowledge the woman's need for safety, but most will accommodate this to some degree. Again, decision-making should be by consensus. This is the client's birth, and she has the ultimate say over what happens to her body. The most powerful words that a client or her partner may use (only in direst need) are, "I do not give my consent for that procedure." These are medico-legal power words that should not be overused: they are directly confrontational and lead to extreme power plays by authorities. However, they are the client's right.

Debriefing

After the birth, it is important that the midwife debrief with the transport physician, both with and without the couple present. The questions we try to answer are: What went right? What can we do differently to improve? What can we learn from this transport? The birthing couple also often need our help in processing the birth. A clear explanation of events and decision-making helps them to be at peace with a transport—something they obviously did not want or plan for.

Sometimes, the things we learn have nothing to do with the medical issues. One of the lay midwives with whom I work learned that when she transports clients to a certain physician, she need say nothing at all while he is in the room; otherwise, he does the opposite of what she suggests.

And sometimes, the bonds between midwife and physician are strengthened merely by the cup of tea and the laughter and tears that are shared after a difficult birth. Now, always, I feel the support and love of my sister midwives as we create our paths within and outside the medical system.

So, in summary: communication, communication, then more communication. The effort often rests with the midwife and her client. But, in time, these efforts will pay off in terms of better relationships with backup physicians and hospital personnel.

Remedies
The Amazing Alfalfa
by Lisa Goldstein, CPM, CNM

MOST PREGNANT WOMEN, like the rest of us, don't get enough green veggies. Alfalfa tablets—a little known, very inexpensive, nutritional supplement—have been of great benefit to my clients and myself for more than 26 years.

The roots of the alfalfa plant, which have been measured to descend more than 125 feet into the earth, bring up many nutrients and micro-nutrients in concentrated amounts. They are very high in both iron and calcium, without interfering with one another as they do in regular (non-whole food) mineral supplements. They are also high in vitamins C, A, E and K, as well as many trace minerals and micro-nutrients.

Many of pregnancy's discomforts are alleviated by the use of alfalfa tablets, including morning sickness, heartburn, constipation and anemia, with its many complications. Alfalfa tablets raise the vitamin K level of pregnant women, reducing postpartum bleeding in both quantity and duration, and they increase the vitamin K stores in newborns, reducing bleeding problems for them as well. Additionally, they support success in lactation because they help increase and sustain milk supply. Alfalfa hay did the same for our goats when we had them.

I have found that most pregnant clients stop taking the extra prenatal iron supplements they are given for the normal mid-trimester hematocrit drop because this form of iron supplement makes them nauseated and/or constipated. Alfalfa tablets frequently help alleviate nausea, almost always relieve constipation, and they bring up the red blood counts in a beneficial way as well. They also seem to help reduce swelling and improve erratic blood sugar levels, perhaps from the nutrient benefit, or perhaps as a secondary gain from the fiber content.

Dosage

To avoid loose bowel movements that some clients—if they have been on a low fiber diet—get from taking too many at a time, I have my clients start slowly. I suggest that they take one alfalfa tablet the first day, then two the second day, and so on until they are taking two after each meal and two before bed. Women with excellent nutrition may not need as many; some with very poor nutritional stores will probably need more. This is the usual number that most women need during pregnancy; in lactation they often can take less.

Over the years many of my clients have told me that the alfalfa tablets have helped them so much, in so many ways, that other family members started taking them too. My husband even takes them when he has digestive upsets. My sons took them when they were teenagers, as they helped with acne (and temperament). I have been told that they have helped people with such diverse health complaints as allergies, arthritis, chronic fatigue, colitis, indigestion, bruising, mouth sores and vaginal infections. As far as I know, no one has had any ill effects from them, only happy results.

I've recently learned alfalfa, like the soybean, is a good source of phytoestrogens. The phytoestrogens act like estrogen in some ways in the body, providing cardiac and cancer-preventative benefits. If the person is lacking in estrogen, the body apparently will use the phytoestrogens as if they were estrogens. If a woman has too much endogenous estrogen on board (which would normally put her at higher breast and endometrial cancer risk), the plant-based helpers protect by binding to the estrogen receptor sites in these places. This may be why women in cultures that eat a lot of soy-based foods have so much less of these forms of cancer than we do. The men have far lower prostate cancer deaths as well.

Contraindications

Because alfalfa tablets are very high in vitamin K, they could be dangerous to take for anyone who needs to be on blood thinners such as Heparin. Always remember that anything we introduce into our bodies, even plants, can have side effects.

Use of alfalfa tablets should be stopped temporarily if one gets a urinary tract infection (due to the possibility of pH changes in the urine) and cut back, at least temporarily, if one gets the "runs." People who have very poor bowel flora may have temporary bouts of gas the first week or so when they start taking them, so they should start at a more gradual pace. I have postpartum moms take a few right after the birth to help with blood loss and bowel movements, then not take any more until the fourth or fifth postpartum day, gradually building back up to about four to eight a day depending on diet and need. They can use oat bran tablets if they need to for bowel function in the meantime. The reason for this is twofold: the degree to which alfalfa promotes lactation can be too much for comfort until engorgement subsides, and newborn jaundice takes longer to go away if the mom is taking alfalfa tablets.

Note

Some pregnant women find that they have a hard time getting the tablets down because they are dry and the smell can bother them. Tell them that they can take out a day's supply and carefully grease the tops and bottoms of them with a little butter or margarine on their index finger and thumb. Gently rub each tablet in between these greasy finger surfaces. The lightly oiled surface will slide down easier, and the aroma will be diminished as well. You can't do many more than a day's worth at a time because they will fall apart from this treatment. Some women have even crushed the tablets and filled gelatin capsules to make them easier to swallow.

I have been told that alfalfa crops are some of the most highly sprayed crops grown, so consider using an organic brand. Read the label to be sure there are no other ingredients in them. Some brands have mint in them, which can antidote homeopathics and may make heartburn worse for some pregnant women because mint can tend to relax the lower esophageal sphincter.

Editor's Note: *This article is extracted from* Using Herbs & Homeopathics in Midwifery Care, *a booklet by Lisa Goldstein, copyright 1998.*

Herbs for Use in Pregnancy, Birth and Postpartum

by Mary Bove, ND, LM

When using herbals with a pregnant woman remember to consider: most herbal constituents will pass through the placenta and reach the fetus; the pregnant body undergoes physiological changes in metabolic processes, which may influence the effect of the herb in the body; you should take extra caution when prescribing in the first trimester; all herbs have the potential to be harmful (use medicinals as medicines); you should choose herbal preparations that complement pregnancy.

Botanical Preparations in Pregnancy

Oral: infusions, tinctures, glycerites, capsules, and tablets
Topical: baths, creams, poultices, peri-wash
Aromatherapy: essential oils

The use of essential oils as massage agents, as additives to baths, or on a tissue as an inhalant can be effective in helping with relaxation and stress reduction, decreasing pain and discomfort in labor, augmenting labor contractions, and facilitating healing and reduction of perineal discomfort during postpartum. A six-month pilot study in British maternity wards showed lavender, clary sage, peppermint and eucalyptus to be among some of the most helpful essential oils studied.

Common Pregnancy Complaints

Constipation: avoid botanical medicines with strong laxative or purgative actions; choose botanicals that act as aperitives, bulking agents, or autonomic visceral relaxants specific for the gastrointestinal tract, such as flax seed, psyllium seed, dandelion (*taraxicum officinalis*), yellow dock (*rumex crispus*), catnip (*nepeta cataria*), and cramp bark (*viburnum opulus*).

Urinary Tract Infection: avoid strong kidney irritants such as *juniperus spp*. Choose botanicals that act as demulcents, urinary astringents: corn silk (*zea mays*), cleavers (*galium aparine*), marshmallow (*althea officinalis*), horsetail (*equisetum spp.*), squawvine (*mitchella repens*), uva ursi (*arctostaphylos*), urinary antiseptics including garlic (*allium sativum*), thyme (*thymus vulgaris*).

Varicosities: e.g., labia. Choose herbs high in bioflavonoids, which act to support connective tissue: crataegus oxyacantha, ginkgo biloba, vaccinium spp.

Hemorrhoids: grated potato and slippery elm poultice for hemorrhoids: 1 medium potato grated, 2-3 teaspoons slippery elm powder. Mix well; form into small patty and place on disturbed area for 10-15 minutes, 1-3 times a day. These may be used on sore or cracked nipples as well.

Postpartum Perineum Fomentation

Calendula flowers (*Calendula officinalis*): used for their vulnerary and anti-inflammatory action.

Basic Herbal Oils and Ointments

Herbal Oil — no cook method
1. All herbs should be chopped or ground (if dried)
2. Put herb into clear glass jar
3. Cover with just enough oil (olive, almond, safflower, sesame) to completely submerge the herb
4. Let sit in a warm sunny place for 10-14 days
5. Strain and filter, discard herb and bottle

Herbal Oil — cook method
1. Prepare herbs and cover with adequate oil
2. Let cook in low oven 110F-150F for 12-15 hours
3. May use slow-cooking crock pot for 12 hours
4. Strain and bottle

Herbal Ointment — general guidelines
1. Use 2 ounces of beeswax to 1 pint oil for ointments
2. Avoid petroleum bases
3. Use salves and oils within a year for best results
4. Store in tightly closed containers in a cool, dark place. Refrigeration is ideal.
5. Mix some essential oils to improve scent, help penetrate the skin and add medicinal qualities.

Directions
1. Grate beeswax
2. Gently heat the prepared herb oil, add in beeswax
3. When wax has melted, pour the hot mixture into containers before it hardens.
4. If adding essential oils, do it when mixture has just been taken off the heat.

Comfrey root (*Symphytum officinalis*): the plant contains a substance that increases cell proliferation, leading to increased tissue repair and growth. It also acts as an astringent, emollient and an anti-inflammatory.

Yarrow flowers: a very effective botanical anti-inflammatory, astringent, anti-microbial and vulnerary. The volatile oil is an important active constituent in these actions.

Rosemary leaves: the actions of antiseptic, astringent and circulatory stimulant make this herb a useful addition to this medicated wash.

Lavender flowers: the flowers contain large amounts of volatile oils, which act as antiseptics, anti-microbials and analgesics. Clinical trial has shown lavender oil as a bath additive to be most effective between the third and fifth days of the postpartum period.

Mix together all of the above ingredients in a jar: use one handful to a pint of boiling water, cover and steep until warm. Use as a sitz bath or in a peri bottle as a perineal wash for cleaning after urination or in sutured areas.

Herbs for Emotional States

by Lisa Goldstein, CPM, CNM

MANY HERBALS HAVE subtle and/or powerful influences on our emotional states. You wouldn't want to become dependent on an herb any more than you would want to be on Valium. During times of stress and emotional struggle, help from an herb might keep you from getting to the place where you felt the need to have a Valium. Some of these need to be taken in tincture form, some can be taken in teas, and some need to be made into infusions to release their properties. Here is a list of a few favorites in alphabetical order to avoid favoritism. This is just a scratch on the surface. To learn more about herbs and their emotional impact read Susun S. Weed's book on menopause titled *Menopausal Years: The Wise Woman Way*.

Chamomile: This is the classic calming herb. It is great for colicky babies or cranky parents. The smell alone imbues relaxation. In tea form it is soothing to the skin and makes a lovely hair rinse.

Catnip: This is one herb I am never without. It makes a good friend at night when you are lying awake exhausted and your brain won't shut up. Even taken at 5 o'clock in the morning when you have to wake an hour later is fine. Tea works fine, though tincture is easier to take when you are half-awake and don't want to get up to make tea. Two drops under the tongue are usually plenty.

Hops: This is the same herb used in making beer. A cup of hops tea can cool your nerves like a glass of beer but without the side effects of alcohol. Try sweetening it with a teaspoon of barley malt syrup or sorghum—chilled in summertime is great. Those with a history of depression should be aware that over time, drinking hops tea could bring about depressive symptoms.

Motherwort: This herb has the reputation of being mildly addicting though most people I've seen use it feel like it was a lifeline for them at a time when they needed it. Under periods of extreme stress, it is an effective nerve soother. In tincture form, take 10-15 drops two to three times daily.

Nettle: Nettle nourishes the body as well as the mind. You can drink all the tea or infusion you want. I like to cook the leaves like greens and use the cooking water chilled as a tea. Nettles is an adrenal toner, a diuretic, a kidney toner, and a red blood cell builder.

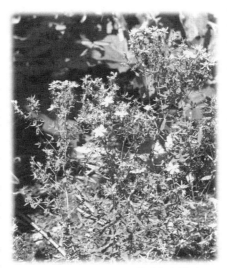

St. John's Wort

Oat Straw: This must be made into an infusion. It is a gentle helper that gradually takes away the harsh edges, the barbs that snag your hurt feelings. I like to make a quart of it at a time and drink it cold, sometimes half and half with juice or other herb tea. Oat straw feeds the nervous system and helps add joy to life.

Senecio Aureus: This herb helps regulate hormonal imbalances. Used in small doses—5-8 drops in water a day—it is effective during the luteal phase (ovulation to menses). It may cause a temporary amplification of symptoms for a month until hormones level out again and also may have a side effect of increasing libido in women. (It does the opposite in men.) Take in the morning or erotic dreams may keep you up at night. Use only the flower tincture, which is, unfortunately, difficult to find since the rest of the plant is considered poisonous. Do not use senecio if you have liver damage, are ill or plan to become pregnant soon.

Skullcap: This is a wonderful herb for calming nervous tension. I use it often for tension headaches.

St. John's Wort (also known as Hypericum): Another wonderful nerve tonic, St. John's wort is especially useful in preventing the lactic acid buildup in the muscles that makes you sore when tense or under strain. Take 2-4 drops of tincture one to three times a day as needed. Not meant for long-term use.

Valerian: This herb is used a lot in Europe as a sleep tonic, a calmative and a treatment for high blood pressure. (Don't use this if you have low blood pressure.) This herb can be habit forming. If needed to help you sleep every night, you should be careful and find other solutions. It will knock you out if you are desperate, however. For folks who don't respond well to catnip, I include this in my herbal mixture that I call Sleep Mix.

Vitex Agnus-castus: The fruit of this bush has properties that help normalize pituitary gland functioning, especially in relation to progesterone production. Many women find this plant very beneficial leading up to and during the menopausal years, especially for calming mood swings. For women it also has the benefit of helping the libido kick in as things are getting normalized.

This is my secret recipe for tension headaches:

In a glass with about an inch of water add:

20 drops of skullcap tincture

3-4 drops of St. John's wort (use 10 drops if menopausal)

5-10 drops of motherwort

This formula usually takes care of a headache in 10 to 20 minutes for me. A friend used to get headaches when she drove on long trips. Since she's started putting this in her water bottle and sipping it all day, she has not had one of those headaches.

Heartburn Treatment Alternatives

by Chris Hafner-Eaton, PhD

ALTHOUGH HEARTBURN IS usually not considered a serious condition during pregnancy, it can be most annoying for the woman. Because some women experience it as an omnipresent condition of pregnancy, caregivers must be prepared for lots of questions about heartburn and have a variety of techniques available to manage it acceptably in different women. Heartburn affects a majority of pregnant women, but certainly not all.

Most women describe a burning sensation in their throat and esophagus, or they may even experience slight regurgitation of stomach acid and food. It may be, in fact, the first time a woman has had this sensation and she may not identify it as heartburn. The underlying causes of this condition are multifaceted and include: general relaxation of the gastrointestinal (GI) tract and peristalsis; the relaxation of specific GI valves/sphincters due to increased progesterone levels and later in pregnancy, due to the fetal position pressing and even kicking into the GI tract.

Common recommendations for heartburn treatment range from the clearly related such as ingesting smaller low-fat meals more frequently, avoiding too much liquid at meals and gaseous foods or carbonated liquids, and working to increase one's exercise. Exercising's effect on heartburn is twofold: it speeds the process of digestion and improves general tone of both voluntary and involuntary muscles. Although the benefits of exercise during pregnancy go far beyond heartburn relief, it is not a viable solution for all. Several practical suggestions that may be made to moms without infringing on their current activity patterns include avoiding tight waistbands and bra bands, sitting and walking with good posture, not lying down flat after a meal, and performing gentle stretching or yoga. Some yoga and tai chi warm-up routines even improve digestion by stimulating the intestines.

Alternatives to commercial or traditional allopathic antacids containing calcium carbonate appeal to many women—especially if they are already ingesting enough calcium through their diet and other natural supplements such as alfalfa or red raspberry leaves. Other women have been advised to intentionally consume non aluminum-based calcium carbonate antacids specifically for the purpose of boosting their calcium intake. In many cases, women need to consume four lozenges at a time up to seven or eight times per day. If a woman is ingesting large amounts of antacids she may be thwarting some of her body's own natural digestive processes, which could make matters worse by slowing down digestion.

One of the most successful approaches to heartburn is to use overall pregnancy tonics such as red raspberry leaf capsules/tincture, alfalfa capsules and nettles infusion. Most midwives will already have recommended these to their patients, although adherence to herbal schedules is not always what it could be. Moms should be started out slowly on tonic herbs if they have not been taking them prior to conception. Start moms out on one capsule (or dropper) three times per day (TID) and work up to three capsules TID. Expectant mothers often need to be reassured that they are not jeopardizing their babies as they would be if they were ingesting large quantities of "medicine"; rather, they should consider these herbs to be true food supplements.

If a woman doesn't want to try the preceding suggestions for whatever reason,
(Continued on next page)

Tips & Tricks

Nausea Aids
My sixth through 12th week were a blur of nausea until I found out about vitamin B-6, ginger and red raspberry leaf. I took a supplement called "Good Morning" made by Solaray. It contains 25 mg vitamin B-6, 325 mg ginger root and 325 mg red raspberry leaf. I highly recommend this supplement.

Jodie Minniear CD, DONA, IN

For nausea during pregnancy, take brewer's yeast in tablet form (10-grain tablets). They're tasteless and odorless with no aftereffects.

Amy (E-News)

Yeast Remedy
For yeast infections I usually recommend 10 drops of teatree oil in 30 drops of a carrier oil such as olive oil, soaked into a cotton tampon. It has remarkable results, but I am cautious about giving this recommendation to anyone postpartum because it is so strong.

C.O. (E-News)

Cervical Scarring
I would recommend that any pregnant woman with cervical scarring take evening primrose oil during the last month of her pregnancy, even applying it directly to her cervix. I had a cervical biopsy done between my third and fourth pregnancies and my labor for my fourth was very painful and long. I rubbed evening primrose oil on my cervix during labor and it seemed to really help things get moving.

Lorrie White (E-News)

Rigid Cervical Os
In a small jar with an eye dropper lid, mix an equal combination of evening primrose oil, spikenard and olive oil to have on hand at births. The mixture is used to lightly massage a rigid os. Shake the container well before using. The eyedropper is a precaution against contamination of the mixture. Do not use this preparation if the woman's membranes are not intact.

Faith Heise, FL

there are herbal treatments to directly address the issue of heartburn. Many women report excellent relief by sipping peppermint tea and chewing papaya-mint tablets. Sucking on peeled fresh ginger (if one can tolerate it) or on candied ginger works for some. In mothers who are exhibiting more complex symptoms such as spastic GI tract, slippery elm (*Ulmus fulva*) will often soothe the GI tract. Slippery elm, in herbalist terms, is a demulcent that soothes irritated mucous membranes. It is also useful as a nutritive tonic to bolster the woman's constitution when in a debilitated state.

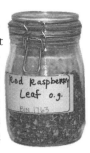

Two herbs used as symptomatic treatments for heartburn include meadowsweet (*Filipendula ulmaria*) and licorice (*Glycyrrhiza glabra*). Both herbs serve us well as anti-inflammatories and reduce stomach acid, but act in different ways in the digestive tract. Licorice reduces the irritation of acid through a buildup of mucous secretion whereas meadowsweet is believed to assist in the proliferation of stomach and intestinal cell reproduction/repair. Caveats exist for both herbs. Avoid the use of licorice with gestational hypertension/toxemia. If the woman has aspirin or salicylate sensitivity, meadowsweet should not be ingested. Ironically, although extended use of aspirin can lead to stomach ulceration, meadowsweet does not exhibit the same negative side effects. Both herbs may be taken internally through a tincture or infusion. If a mother is close to term and experiences gas as well as heartburn, then fennel should be considered a treatment possibility. Fennel is considered a strong laxative and uterine stimulant, so its use earlier in pregnancy is not desirable.

Treating heartburn symptomatically with herbs is less than ideal because we fall into the same trap as when using allopathic medicine: chasing symptoms around the body. It is far better to holistically manage the pregnant woman as a synergistic being with many interacting systems. When we fail to recognize this or choose to ignore it and resort to treating symptoms only, for example, by using commercial antacids, we must acknowledge that there will be counter-reactions in the body.

Homeopathy: What It Is and How to Apply It

by Lisa Goldstein, CPM, CNM

A BASIC UNDERSTANDING of homeopathy is essential to making good decisions about its use. First of all, homeopathy is not the same thing as herbal medicine. Although most of the remedies are made from plant sources, that is only one similarity. Homeopathic remedies can be made from mineral and even some animal sources as well. The remedies are made in a way that dilutes them in a specific, sequential way. They become so diluted that there is little of the original substance left that a lab would find. This is one of the reasons that these remedies are so safe. It is also what makes homeopathy mysterious to most scientific minds. How do they work then? Though many theories exist, no one actually really knows. The great thing is that they work.

Because they are so complex, it is much more difficult to learn about homeopathy. There is not just one remedy for a cough, for example. There may be 20 or more remedies for a complaint, depending on the specific symptoms. Having an excellent book or several books on homeopathy is essential if you are to find the perfect remedy. This may be annoying and may seem to take a lot of effort at first. Gradually, as you learn remedies and see results for your family, however, you

(Continued on next page)

Tips & Tricks

Miscarriage
When a woman is miscarrying, I give her angelica tincture once I see that enough tissue has passed or the fetus is out so that the placenta will be expelled intact. I have her take one full dropperful of tincture in a small glass of warm water every 10 to 15 minutes. I stop giving it if the woman throws up.

Jill Cohen, OR

Postpartum Blues & Breast Milk
My midwives were herbalists with lots of experience under their belts. One of them made me a wonderful herbal cocktail that is delicious and effective for not only postpartum blues but for fortifying breast milk. I make a tea from red clover, great for purifying the blood and helping improve breast milk; lemon balm, which works wonderfully for lifting the spirits; red raspberry leaf, which helps the uterine walls contract so that the uterus can shrink back down to size; and nettles, which contains vitamin K, important for clotting. Nettles also is a good source of iron, which is important for breastfeeding babies. I steep a teaspoon of each per cup of tea for about five minutes. It is best fresh!

Grace (E-News)

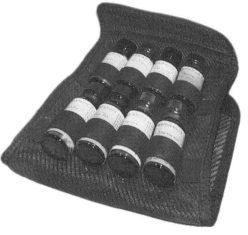

Tips & Tricks

Pinworm Remedies

Before medications for pinworms were developed, gentian violet was taken internally for 10 days to kill the worms. It cannot be used internally in pregnancy, but it does raise the possibility of external use at the anus to kill emerging worms. Some naturopaths prescribe spigelia for pinworms. It is safe to use in pregnancy. Others suggest ingestion of pumpkin seeds and garlic for a period of 10 days to two weeks. It is important for all family members to be treated, and this includes bathing every morning to wash away ova that have been deposited outside the anus. Snug fitting underwear and regular hand washing as well as washing of bed sheets will also reduce reinfestation.

Maryl Smith (E-News)

Pumpkin seeds as a remedy for pinworms is very effective. It will kill them and eliminate them from the body. I don't have specific advice other than to eat pumpkin seeds until the problem resolves, and I'd advise eating them until three weeks after that to ensure there are no hatching visitors. A quarter cup three times a day seems like a reasonable amount.

Beth Germano (E-News)

Labor Preparation Aid

We start our moms on "Labor Prep" tincture at 36 weeks. It consists of:
- 2 parts partridgeberry
- 1 part each, black haw/black cohosh
- 1/2 part helonias

Take 1/2 tsp twice a day and 1 tsp before bed. At 40 weeks we add one part spikenard and increase the dose to 1 tsp three times a day. No one has gone more than seven days past the estimated due date since we started the protocol this year.

Anon. (E-News)

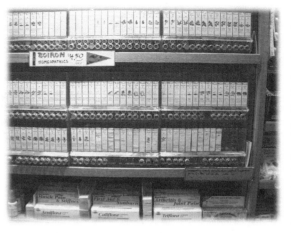

won't mind the effort involved in tracking down the right remedy. Homeopathy is not a substitute for medical care but a simple way of treating common health problems that are not medical emergencies. It can save you lots of trips to the drugstore.

You should usually start with a few common remedies and your first book. When you get comfortable seeing results, you may want to buy a kit of remedies. Then you'll want a more extensive book. Though the greater field of homeopathy may seem overwhelming at first, try not to grow discouraged. The first time you wake up in the middle of the night coughing and find the right remedy that gives you a decent night's sleep, you'll know why people are so happy with homeopathy.

How Do I Take a Remedy?

Pour a few pellets into the cap of the bottle and drop them under your tongue to dissolve. If you are using the liquid solutions, drop two drops under your tongue. Be sure not to touch the remedies or the dropper tip to anything. You need to have a clean mouth when taking remedies, which means you shouldn't eat, drink or smoke for 15-20 minutes before and after taking the remedy. If you are experiencing an emergency condition, however, don't wait to take the remedy, and repeat the dosage every few minutes, if necessary.

How Often Do I Take the Remedy?

If you are seeing a practitioner, the practitioner will tell you exact directions. If you are self-treating, generally you take the remedy only when the symptoms are present. If your symptoms persist, you may want to try a higher potency of the same remedy. If you get an "aggravation" (an overstimulation of the healing process: stronger symptoms rather than improvement), stop taking the remedy until this subsides and contact your practitioner. If the symptoms are particularly troubling, you can always "antidote" them (see below).

Antidoting Your Remedy:

There are some things that can antidote a remedy; that is, they usurp the effectiveness of the remedy. The most common antidotes are: coffee (in any form), mints (toothpaste, gums, etc.), camphor and tea tree oil. For some people eucalyptus and menthol also antidote remedies. For others, not even coffee negates a remedy. Electromagnetic fields and recreational drugs such as steroids can also negate the effects of homeopathics. Homeopathics will not interfere with allopathic (prescription) medicines, however. You will have to learn what works for you.

Homeopathics work on infants and animals as well as grown-ups. You will probably hear some people insist that homeopathic remedies work as a placebo because of the minuscule amounts of formula in them. I leave it up to you, the reader. What do you think?

Black Cohosh: Uterine Effects

by Cindy Belew, CNM, Herbalist

Several herbs have a variety of effects on uterine activity—black haw, cramp bark, blue cohosh, cottonroot, helonias, false unicorn, lobelia, motherwort, partridgeberry, shepherd's purse, trillium, vitex, chasteberry and wild yam. In this volume we will look at one of the more known herbs: black cohosh.

Black Cohosh

Botanical Name: *Cimicifuga racemosa*
Preparation and Dosage: Fresh or dry root tincture, 10-25 drops up to 4x a day; or capsules, "00" size, 1-2 three times daily.

History of Use

Late 19th century physicians such as the Eclectics considered black cohosh to be a "remedy par excellence to stimulate normal functional activity of the uterus and ovaries" throughout the reproductive life cycle. They used it to "reduce unpleasant sensation and false pains in the pregnant uterus, and aid true pains" and for pelvic pains, soreness and backache during pregnancy. They reported that when used regularly at the end of pregnancy "it will render labor easier and quicker, and give a better getting up." The author states this was based upon his observations of 32 years of practice and the "like experience of other good observers."

Knox, an Eclectic physician, presented a paper before the Chicago Gynecological Society describing his use of black cohosh in combination with sarsaparilla in 160 women during the last four weeks of pregnancy to prepare them for labor. Under its use, he had found the average duration of the first stage reduced from 17 hours to 6 hours and a quarter, and that of the second stage from three hours to an hour and three quarters, in primiparae; that of the first stage from 12 hours to three hours, and that of the second stage from an hour to 27 minutes, in multiparae. From his observations he had concluded that the drug had a

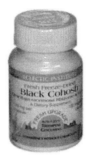

positive sedative effect on parturient women, quieting reflex irritability, nausea, pruritis and insomnia; that it mitigated, and often altogether abolished, the neuralgic cramps and irregular pains of the first stage; that it relaxed the soft parts, thus facilitating labor and diminishing the risks of laceration; that it increased the energy and the rhythm of the pains in the second stage; and that, like ergot, it maintained a better contraction of the uterus after delivery.

Herbalists use black cohosh as an antispasmodic in areas other than reproductive health as well, including rheumatic pain. It is considered specific for pain of a dull, heavy, aching nature, or for soreness or bruised feeling in the muscles, not for sharp pain (wild yam is specific for sharp pain).

Felter stated that black cohosh is "the ideal regulator of uterine contractions during labor, an "excellent partus preparator" and "a diagnostic agent to differentiate between spurious and true labor pains, the latter being increased, while the former are dissipated under its use."

Research

Isolated constituents of black cohosh have peripheral vasodilatory and hypotensive effects in animals (Leung & Foster, 1996). Researchers reporting on human studies have stated, "In man, this drug (isolated constituent of black cohosh) has no hypotensive effect, though its peripheral vasodilatory is evident" (Genazzani & Sorrentino, 1962, p. 545).

Actions

Uterine tonic and relaxing nervine. Warming, increases peripheral blood flow and disperses congestion.

Indications

- Alone or in formula with other herbs during the last month of pregnancy to prepare for labor.
- Pelvic discomfort, excessive uterine activity or tone, false labor during the last month of pregnancy.
- To augment or initiate labor contractions.
- Dull, achy heavy feeling in pelvis or legs.
- Postpartum uterine subinvolution with heavy, aching pain.

Cautions

Do not use before 36 weeks' gestation. Newell (1996) cautions to avoid excessive doses but does not indicate what constitutes an excessive dose. Moore (1996) notes that large doses can induce a frontal headache and that it is a central nervous system depressant in some persons.

Other: Black cohosh has a number of uses in gynecology. In clinical studies black cohosh has been efficacious in relieving various symptoms of menopause. A metabolite of black cohosh is perceived by the pituitary as estrogen metabolites, suppressing the release of luteinizing hormone.

Sources

Felter, F. H. (1993). *The Eclectic Materia Medica, Pharmacology and Therapeutics*. Portland, Ore.: Eclectic Medical Publications.

Genazzani, E., and Sorrentino, L. (1962). Vascular action of acteina: Active constituent of Actea Racemosa L. *Nature* 194: 544-5.

Moore, M. (1996). *Herbal Tinctures in Clinical Practice*. 3rd ed. Southwest School of Botanical Medicine.

Newell, C., Anderson, L. A., and Phillipson, J. D. (1996). *Herbal Medicines: A Guide for Health-Care Professionals*. London: The Pharmaceutical Press.

Scudder, J. M. (1996). Uterine remedies. *The Eclectic Medical Journals: The John M. Scudder Organ Remedies, 1892-1892*, 2(6): 73-74.

Bottoms and Births

by Lisa Goldstein, CPM, CNM

ANYONE WHO GREW up in the mountains where I live probably knows about yellow root. It's an old remedy for sour stomach, nausea, carsickness and indigestion, and can be applied directly to mouth sores. The boiled root makes a nastily bitter tea. I made a tincture with it to see if one could use less of the nasty stuff and get the same results. The results were great! Usually, only one drop is needed. Placing it under the tongue makes the taste more tolerable, and the herb is absorbed directly by the mucus membrane and gets into your system quicker.

Green Balm

This is a great remedy for painful hemorrhoids. Mix plantain leaves with witch hazel in a blender, strain and then dilute the result with a little water. Keep the mixture cold for best results. On a mini-pad, it can be applied directly to the needy area, or pour it into a jar of cotton balls to be used for cleansing. This is great for sore bottoms, especially if the cottonballs are chilled; it works even better frozen in severe situations, like right after a birth. Round the balm-moistened cottonballs and freeze on a plate. Now put one balm ball right where it will do the most good. Change when changing peri-pad or as needed.

Comfrey Salve

This herbal—easy to make and a useful first-aid treatment for many skin problems—is actually famous for using on sore nipples. The comfrey leaf has allantoin, which promotes regeneration of epithelial (skin) cells. You need only a tiny amount to help itchy bug bites, as well as sunburn and poison ivy, dry red skin, sore nipples and sore baby bottoms. Submerge clean, dry comfrey leaves in a good quality oil for six to eight weeks. Strain, then heat to kill bacteria. Thicken with beeswax and/or paraffin and pour into small jars. It doesn't smell very good because comfrey is a very gassy plant, but it is wonderful stuff.

Arnica Massage Oil

No herbal list would be complete without reference to arnica. It often is like an answer to prayer for muscle, joint pain, bruising and any kind of tissue trauma. Rub it on or in, and the pain is relieved. Try it during perineal massage, both in prenatal time (getting the skin stretched and ready) and during the birth itself. I once used olive oil during births, but arnica works much better. It seems to make perineums "feel like silk," as a friend says. The books say do not use arnica oil on broken skin, but I have no problems with it during a birth. There has also been concern that the oil weakens latex gloves. Change to new ones if using arnica longer than 10 minutes, to reduce chances of breakdown (oil can break down latex's integrity). I can truthfully say I've never had gloves break down due to arnica oil—and I have saved some bottoms!

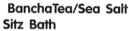
photo by Suzanne Arms

Arnica Solution

I also want to mention arnica solution, a homeopathic form of arnica. If you don't have arnica solution already made up at a birth, you can make up a quickie form by dissolving some pellets in clean water in a jar or an unused perineal squirt bottle. Dribble a little of this in the center of the absorbent side of six peri-pads (if using the regular solution, first dampen with two or three teaspoons of water and then drop about eight drops of the arnica solution on this area). Put these pads in the freezer (damp side up, or they'll stick). Use them as the first pads you use after a birth. They will make a huge difference in comfort and work magic on swelling. The next morning, mom is usually swollen again, so make another one or two pads in advance, to use then. Mom can use a few drops (or pellets) in the peri bottle for rinsing when urinating, if there is any pain during the process.

Arnica can be given by mouth as well and will make a dramatic change in the swelling, bruising and pain. Use arnica on 4x4 gauze squares if you prefer. These are helpful on the sore little baby bottoms of breech-birth babies.

BanchaTea/Sea Salt Sitz Bath

I learned about bancha tea from a client in the 1960s She was from Japan and said its use was customary there. You use about 11 cups of bancha tea (or twig tea, a green tea from Japan). Put this tea in a pot with about three quarts of water and simmer for 10 minutes. Strain it and add about 1 cup sea salt (save the tea leaves). Put this strained tea into a sitz bath while warm (sometimes, if swelling is severe, cooler tea works better) and sit in it. If it bums, there's too much salt; dilute with water. Stay in the sitz bath until it cools. Use the tea to make another batch, but simmer this time for 20 minutes. Simmer a third batch for 30 minutes. Each time, be sure to use a healing salt, not one from the supermarket (it will bum). Most who have used this treatment have felt that healing was expedited, especially if stitches were present. I used this especially for first-time mothers, but since I'm using more arnica in the last few years, both by mouth and as a topical oil during the birth, I have not needed bancha tea and sea salt sitz bath. Bottoms are just in better shape. Still, it's good to know about if you need it for someone and have no arnica.

Urinary Tract Infections

by Lisa Goldstein, CPM, CNM

How can you tell if you have a urinary tract infection, or UTI? The most common symptoms are: the urge to "go" all the time; a feeling of fullness, even if you just "went"; a burning feeling during peeing (it may feel "hot"); sharp, strong pains in the bladder area; and pain in the low back on either side in the kidney area.

While pregnant, it is possible to have a UTI with little or no symptoms. If not treated, a urinary tract infection can be dangerous to you and your baby during pregnancy. Pregnant women should heed the following suggestions to minimize the risk of acquiring a UTI.

First things first: after you've gone to the bathroom, pay attention! Do you wipe from the back to the front? If you do, you are wiping bacteria from around your rectum into the vaginal area. This can cause vaginal infections or irritations and/or urinary tract infections. Learn to wipe front to back.

Secondly, do you hold your urine when you feel you need to go? Research has determined it is unsafe to hold your pee. If you feel the need to pee, do so. Holding it can cause an accumulation of bacteria in the bladder that increases one's risk of acquiring a UTI.

While pregnant, a woman is more prone to UTIs due to increased pressure, difficulty in fully emptying her bladder and more dampness in the area. Because a pregnant woman develops more lubrication to help her baby slide out, this may attract bacteria, especially when one wears tight clothes that cut off circulation. Think of the bladder of a pregnant woman as a pitcher that has trouble fully emptying due to the pressure of the baby. If it gets more than 12 drops in it, the bladder feels like it's going to rupture from the pressure. But after peeing, it feels full again in 20 minutes—partly because it didn't actually get emptied.

One way to get a few more drops out is to stand and tilt forward, gently lifting the belly to the right and then to the left. Each time you'll get a little more out by "tipping the pitcher." This may sound silly at first, but the relief gained is worth it.

Cranberry juice has a unique ability to attach itself to bacteria in the urine and pull them out of the bladder. It is a good idea in pregnancy—or if you are unusually prone to UTIs—to drink a quart of cranberry juice a week. If you don't like it plain, try the cranberry/raspberry or cranberry/blueberry varieties. If avoiding sugar, unsweetened cranberry juice is available at health food stores. Though more expensive, it is concentrated and can be diluted with water or other fruit concentrates to match your taste. Cranberry capsules are also available.

During lovemaking bacteria can get rubbed into the urethra, migrate up into the bladder and cause UTI. After lovemaking, be sure to pee within fifteen minutes because this will rinse unwanted intruders out of there. Also be sure your honey has washed his hands before you go to bed since hands are a common carrier of infection. Be especially careful of contact around the anus. Remember the wiping lesson?

Some women have discovered that Nutrasweet Artificial Sweetener makes their urethra hurt. There have not yet been studies to determine whether Nutrasweet increases UTIs, so pay attention to this possibility. Finally, if you are taking prescription medicines, be sure you are taking them as directed. Taking only a part of the recommended dosage may cause unknown side effects, which might lead to a UTI.

If you do succumb to a urinary tract infection, see your health care provider. But by following these safeguards and prevention strategies, a pregnant woman should be able to moderately guard herself against the discomfort and safety concerns of a urinary tract infection.

Tips & Tricks
Preterm labor

I have had excellent results with the following: 1500 mg calcium and 750 mg magnesium daily. Also include six tablets of alfalfa daily, and nettles. If contractions come on and there are more than normal Braxton Hicks, have the woman take black haw tincture—usually 10 to 20 drops, one dose; if she is still contracting in 20 to 30 minutes, repeat the dosage. Combine this with bed rest. She also needs to drink plenty of water daily (more than she wants). Of course, she should be checked by a doctor if the herb doesn't stop contractions.

Linda Myers, CPM (E-News)

I use several different methods, depending on the woman. But I have had good luck with all of these: Benadryl, cell salt (magnesium phosphate), Rescue Remedy, valerian, vodka, checkup for urinary infection (get it treated), and a moist heating pad on mom's lower abdomen, right above her pubic hair. Also, if baby is breech or in another malposition that is stimulating the cervix, I give pulsatilla to get the baby moved. I also use bed rest with baby's head off the cervix. Calcium with magnesium also may work. Humor and prayer can work well, too.

S.H. (E-News)

A doctor in the town where I work (I am an RN, not a CNM) advises his patients to drink one or two glasses of red wine if they are having contractions. I do not know the efficacy of this, but I do know we don't get very many of his patients coming to the hospital in preterm labor.

M. Farney (E-News)

I have had very good luck with the herb vibernum opulus (cramp bark). I use a dropperful of tincture in water as needed (up to every five minutes) to stop contractions (in addition to rest and fluids, of course). I also used the tincture—three times daily for the first trimester—to prevent miscarriage.

Margy Porter (E-News)

Herbal Allies for Childbirth

by Kathryn Cox

CHILDBIRTH BRINGS UP a wide range of emotions during the final month of pregnancy. One can feel ecstasy at the miracle of birth, as well as the fear of pain and of self-doubt. The atmosphere you create for the birth is very important. Choose a birthplace where you will feel the most comfortable and secure. This should be a place where you can bring any special items that will enhance your birth experience—music, photos, gemstones, fresh flowers, a camera and friends. This is truly a time of transformation, and there are many ways to prepare for it. Childbirth classes teach breathing techniques for natural pain relief and focus. It can be helpful to learn which acupressure points relieve back labor pain and help open the cervix.

Herbs are also a great birthing ally. Used successfully by midwives for years to ease labor pain and reduce the need for drug intervention, herbs also progress a stalled labor, slow bleeding, calm anxiety, provide focus, and give renewed strength and nourishment.

When I was pregnant with my first child, I decided to have a homebirth. Since we lived in the mountains in Colorado, far from a hospital, my husband and I drove to my midwife's home in town when I went into labor. This way we were closer to a hospital in case of any unforeseen emergency. A long, intense labor gave me plenty of opportunity to use my pain relieving tinctures of cramp bark and skullcap. We drove to the hospital when, after more than 30 hours of labor, I had dilated to only three centimeters. Now hooked up to fetal monitors and Pitocin, my cervix still would not dilate. Our first daughter was born by cesarean. Her head was tilted back and the umbilical cord wrapped around her neck three times. The doctor told me that she would have suffocated had she ever entered the birth canal.

I was grateful for the herbs that helped me through the long labor and for the medical expertise that saved our lives. When I returned home from the hospital I put mashed comfrey leaves on the cesarean cut, and I am happy to say that today I have no visible scar.

I was confident that I could have a successful vaginal birth with my second child, but my husband was not willing to try a homebirth again. The local hospital had beautiful birthing rooms where I could bring my ritual objects, and where I was encouraged to use my herbal tinctures during labor when I needed them. Soon after the birth of our second daughter I took a combination tincture of cramp bark, motherwort and raspberry leaf to prevent any afterbirth cramping, give me the emotional support that I needed, and slow after-birth bleeding. I

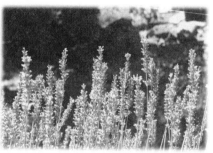

Lavender

continued to take this for three days.

Our second daughter had a heart defect that was discovered the day after she was born. She went through a series of tests for days, and the sitz bath and homeopathic arnica were invaluable to me, as I was able to walk and sit comfortably through the many appointments.

With my third pregnancy I was two weeks overdue. After consulting with my nurse midwife, I took a dose of blue cohosh tincture. Six hours later I went into labor. When we arrived at the hospital, once again I was dilated to only three centimeters. But in less than an hour of soaking in the hot tub with my oldest daughter pushing the pressure points on my lower back, I was ready to push. Our third daughter was soon born. The birth went very quickly. I walked and squatted as we waited for the placenta to expel. The midwife tried herbs, and then Pitocin, but nothing worked. Unknown to her, the placenta had adhered to the uterine wall on my previous cesarean scar, and I was hemorrhaging internally. The warm blood came gushing out as the doctor on call prepared to do an emergency hysterectomy to stop the bleeding. I had my husband squeeze a dropperful of fresh shepherd's purse tincture into my mouth. Almost instantly the bleeding "miraculously" stopped, and an incredulous doctor was able to do a D & C to remove the placenta instead of the previously planned hysterectomy.

As you prepare for this very special time, remember these herbal allies. Just as they helped me, they can also help you minimize the pain, help promote rapid healing after the birth and reduce the need for any unnecessary drug intervention.

Tinctures, Tonics, Oils and Teas

Tinctures are an easy way to use herbs during labor. Tinctures are already prepared when the need for them arises, and they work very quickly. They are made by combining herbs in alcohol and water to extract the active ingredients. After a period of time this liquid is strained and bottled. Herbal drops can then be taken in a small amount of water to dissipate the alcohol, or used directly from the dropper bottle. I mixed my own tinctures, but they are readily available in natural food stores.

Raspberry leaf (*Rubus idaeus*), best known as the premiere uterine tonic, can be taken throughout pregnancy and labor. Just as a runner prepares his or her leg muscles before a marathon, raspberry leaf strengthens the uterine muscles so they will work more efficiently during contractions. Raspberry leaf also helps expel the placenta after birth, slow after-birth bleeding and increase breastmilk.

(Continued on next page)

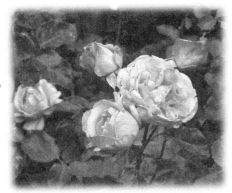
Rose

For convenience prepare a tea or ice chips ahead of time to sip or suck on during labor. Add chamomile (*Matricaria recutita*) for a relaxing effect.

Skullcap (*Scutellaria lateriflora*), chamomile and catnip (*Nepeta cataria*) tinctures, as well as homeopathic chamomile and St. John's wort (*Hypericum perforatum*), work well to relieve tension and ease labor pain. As the name implies, cramp bark (*Viburnum opulus*) eases uterine cramping during labor, as well as the pains after birth. When the ups and downs and feelings of anxiety seem overwhelming, motherwort (*Leonurus cardiaca*) is the herb to use. Rescue Remedy, a Bach flower remedy, also helps one to refocus when under stress. The baby can also benefit with drops of Rescue Remedy on the wrists or forehead. And you can use aromatherapy inhalers made with specific essential oil combinations that give emotional focus, clarity and rejuvenation.

Two tinctures that many midwives use are blue cohosh (*Caulophyllum thalictroides*) and shepherd's purse (*Capsella bursa pastoris*). Blue cohosh brings on labor when the baby is overdue and should not be used before the last month of pregnancy. And during a long, stalled labor, blue cohosh makes contractions more efficient and revitalizes an irritable mother-to-be. Shepherd's purse works immediately to stop postpartum hemorrhaging. But in order for it to work most effectively make sure the tincture is made with fresh, not dried, shepherd's purse.

Relieve back labor pain and tension with a massage using an oil made with herbs such as chamomile, rose (*Rosa*), calendula (*Calendula officinalis*) and lavender (*Lavendula*). You can also add an essential oil with a scent that you find comforting. Perineal massage is helpful before labor and as the baby crowns to prevent tearing, ease any swelling and lessen the sensation of burning. An herbal oil of comfrey (*Symphytum officinalis*) or St. John's wort works well for this. And if you do tear or have an episiotomy, this oil will promote rapid healing.

Homeopathic arnica pills reduce the swelling of bruised perineal muscles after birth. Arnica should be taken in homeopathic form only, not as an herbal tincture, because it may prevent clotting. Arnica salve should never be put on a bleeding wound for the same reason. A sitz bath brings immediate relief to swollen membranes and slows bleeding. Look for a mixture that contains a combination of herbs such as comfrey, yarrow (*Achillea millefolium*), uva ursi (*Arctostaphylos uva-ursi*), witch hazel (*Hamamelis virginica*), goldenseal (*Hydrastus canadensis*) or garlic (*Allium sativum*).

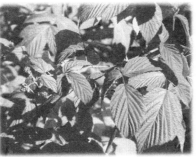
Red Raspberry

To use, pour one gallon of boiling water over one ounce of herbs. Cover and steep for 20 minutes. Strain the strong infusion into a shallow tub or a sitz bath pan specifically made to sit in on the toilet. Squirt a strong comfrey tea from a bottle as you urinate, to prevent burning and also aid in perineal healing.

Chances are you will not need all of these items at the birth. But I have learned, after experiencing three very different births, that it is worth it to be herbally prepared for anything that may happen.

Tips & Tricks

Vaginal Swab

The vagina should have an acid pH, but douching should never be done during pregnancy. If a woman is having symptoms of yeast because of a pH imbalance, have her mix two teaspoons of white vinegar and one cup water; store in a jar with a tight lid to avoid evaporation. She can wet three to four Q-tips in the solution and swab her vagina. This may be repeated several times a day if needed.

This can be done after treatment for yeast infections to prevent recurrences, at times when a woman has a lot of discharge with no other symptoms, and after intercourse (semen has a base pH). If the woman complains of external itchiness, she can spray or pour the solution over her genitals.

Unknown

Digestion Aid (fat eater)

Take in the morning before breakfast or before a heavy meal, especially one that includes meat. Ingredients: 1-2 tsp. lecithin, 1 tsp. honey, 2 tsp. good cider vinegar. Mix all in a cup of hot water; if left to sit a few mintues it will dissolve a little. Often I need to add another half-cup of water if I've made it too strong. This is a wonderful digestive aid.

Maryanne Vella, NZ, (E-News)

Nettles

I encourage all my clients to drink 16-32 oz. of nettles tea every day. For women who just cannot drink this tea or in that quantity, I suggest taking the herb in capsule form (two caps, three times a day).

Nettles tea is a superior natural thirst quencher, high in Vitamin K, iron and important anti-oxidants. Mixed with other woman-friendly herbs such as oat straw, red raspberry leaf and red clover, these herbs support the expanding blood volume and tone the uterus. It is a wonderful and refreshing beverage hot or cold. Taken during labor, it provides all important, blood clotting Vitamin K for mother and baby. After the baby comes, it continues to refresh the mother, and helps increase milk production.

Kim Mosny, CPM, TN

Traditional Chinese Medicine for Hemorrhage

by Valerie Hobbs, Midwife, Doctor of Chinese Medicine

I CAN STILL remember the day it dawned on me that the practice of American midwifery is based on Western medicine.

I had long integrated alternative disciplines into my practice, which I thought made my practice holistic. I truly believed that to use herbs, a bit of homeopathy, visualizations, prevention and non-intervention meant I had somehow transformed the medical model of care on which some midwifery seemed to be based. That was, until the blue cohosh didn't work.

I had long been certain the only reason herbs didn't work was because they were either not prepared properly or not treated properly. Perhaps the herbs were old. Maybe the tinctures were decanted on the new moon. Perhaps the gatherer hadn't meditated enough over the plant. I sought to avoid those potential problems by living on the land, hunting my own herbs, leaving the grandmother plant while making some kind of offering to the plants I collected, harvesting at the right moon cycle, and preparing my own tinctures. I had the most righteous blue cohosh tincture in the universe—I knew it would work.

For Debbie, it worked like a charm. It was an herbal wonder, and I felt I had a handle on hemorrhage. Then Connie bled, and the blue cohosh didn't make a bit of difference. What was going on?

Later a friend asked me what kind of hemorrhage it had been—bright blood, dark blood? She suggested that maybe Chinese herbs would have been more direct. Someone else suggested that other substances from Chinese medicine could have been used.

So came the day I realized that midwifery is based on Western medicine. My peer review group had arranged an educational seminar with a local practitioner of Traditional Chinese Medicine (TCM). He talked about the popularized use of moxa that was used for mother roasting. He explained that there were certain times it shouldn't be used, like when there was bright red bleeding postpartum that seemed rather profuse or prolonged, red tongue, red cheeks, fever—and he called these symptoms signs of "heat."

Then it hit me: in the Western world we name a condition, try to translate it into an anatomy and physiology model, and call it done. Midwives may bring in alternative methods for treating it, but the basic theory concentrates on dissection and compartmentalization. Herbology follows the same line of reasoning—plants are described as lactagogues, emmenagogues, febrifuges, diaphoretics and oxytocics, for example. In Chinese medicine, other symptoms are considered. These symptoms may not have anything to do with the immediate anatomy and physiology of the Western condition, yet they are truly "whole-istic." Instead of treating a condition in a person, you treat the person who has the condition.

While herbal medicine is well developed in the West, it is more developed in the East. The Eastern tradition follows 2,000 years of uninterrupted, unchallenged study and knowledge, whereas the Western tradition is based on a few hundred years of knowledge that precariously survived concerted attacks upon on herbalists during the Dark Ages in Europe. Even though we midwives know the pitfalls of relying on Western medicine as a model, our herbal medicine is based on the Western model of diagnosis and treatment. If we recognize the limitations of Western medicine as it applies to women's health, why do we embrace only Western-based herbology?

Basic TCM Theory

Basically, traditional Chinese medicine (TCM) boils down to three aspects: the theory of organs and channels, the theory of vital substances and the theory of pathogens (translated literally as "evils").

Even though TCM organs have names that are translated into English using the same organ names as used in the English language (lung, liver, spleen, and so on), TCM organs are functional rather than anatomical. The functions of TCM organs are not at all the same as Western functions. For instance, the spleen is responsible for "transformation and transportation of qi," which is roughly equivalent to the Western function of digestion. The TCM spleen has no lymphatic function, as it does in the Western modality.

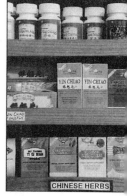
CHINESE HERBS

Vital substances are qi, blood, essence and fluids. Qi is loosely translated as "energy," although this is not an exact match in language, as the ancient Chinese had no word for energy as distinct from matter. Qi is an energetic principle, but it is also matter that exists in more dense and more rare forms; it is the substrate of movement and is movement at the same time. Qi has certain functions—notably to warm, to activate (meaning all physiology and metabolism), to protect against pathogenic "evils," to transform (to change qi into other vital substances, to form sweat and urine, and so on), and to contain. The function of qi in containment means that it is the qi that "holds" or "contains" the blood within the vessels and prevents loss of fluids through abnormal sweating.

Blood is formed from essential qi derived from food by the spleen. Blood is moved throughout the body by qi. The function of blood is to nourish the whole body. A pathology of blood, called blood stasis, is caused by generalized impairment of the smooth movement of blood, a localized stagnation of blood in the vessels, or a local accumulation

(Continued on next page)

of extravasated blood. Stasis can block the normal flow of qi and blood and cause the blood to further extravasate, and a hemorrhage occurs.

By combining the theories of organs and vital substances, one can then see if a function of the spleen is to hold blood in the vessels (accomplished by spleen qi), and if the spleen qi fails to function, it results in extravasation of blood, and a hemorrhage occurs.

The third aspect of TCM is the presence of pathogens or "evils." These evils were observed in the environment and were described as causing certain signs and symptoms as they invaded the body. Sometimes these evils are generated by disharmony in the function of organs. Most notable in our discussion of hemorrhage is the fire evil. Fire can scorch the blood and cause frenetic movement of blood that causes the blood to overflow the channels, and hemorrhage occurs.

Patterns That Cause Hemorrhage

All conditions in TCM are delineated by the pattern that presents. The patterns that cause hemorrhage are qi vacuity, blood stasis and blood heat.

Qi vacuity: This term means that the qi is "empty" or vacuous. It is exhausted in such a way that it can no longer maintain its function; in the case of hemorrhage, it can no longer contain blood. A hemorrhage due to qi vacuity can be profuse or a slow, thin trickle. The blood is usually a watery or pale kind of red. Other symptoms of qi vacuity are weakness; general lack of strength; shallow, pale complexion; feeble voice; spontaneous sweating; aversion to chills; a pale tongue; and a weak, thin pulse. A kind of qi vacuity that further complicates a hemorrhage is when the qi is "sinking." In this case the qi is "empty" but also fails to ascend, causing the blood to "fall" in a hemorrhage. The bleed is similar to that seen in qi vacuity, with the addition of a feeling of heaviness in the abdomen, or actual organ prolapse (rectal, cervical or uterine).

Blood stasis: Hemorrhage due to blood stasis is characterized by a dark red-purple to black color with clots that can be small or large, by fixed pain, by a dull, dark facial complexion (especially around the lips), by a tongue that is purplish or has purplish or ecchymotic areas to it, and by what is known as a rough pulse, meaning that it is slightly irregularly irregular. (Pulse distinction takes time to learn so practitioners should not use it diagnostically unless they have some TCM experience.)

Blood heat: A hemorrhage from heat in the blood is profuse, bright red or thick bright red. Heat can manifest as a repletion (meaning "full" heat) or as vacuity heat (meaning "empty" heat), so the accompanying signs and symptoms can be a sensation of heat, red face or red cheeks, thirst, dry mouth and tongue, irritability, dark urine, a red tongue or just red at the tip, and a rapid full or rapid fine pulse (rapid in TCM is more than 90 bpm).

Herbs for Hemorrhage

After the cause of hemorrhage is recognized and differentiated, herbs can be used to act on the cause. In TCM, herbs are described in terms of categories with certain actions such as blood quickeners, wind-heat resolvers, qi boosters and so on. Herbs can also have a taste. Pungent herbs are usually dispersing, sweet herbs are supplementing, and bitter herbs are cooling. Herbs have property, which is their temperature. They have direction: dispersing, moving up and out, contracting, moving in and down, descending and ascending. And finally they have functions, some primary and some secondary.

Information on Western herbs in TCM language is a relatively new phenomenon, occurring in this generation only. Since TCM language has been refined for more than a hundred generations, one must understand that there may be some inaccuracies in the newer descriptions. With this in mind, following are some descriptions of Western herbs that are familiar friends of midwives. Some of these are known in TCM, and where this is the case, a name is given in the pinyin spelling of Chinese words. If no name appears in pinyin, the herb is a Western one.

(Continued on next page)

Tips & Tricks

Genital Herpes

If a client experiences an outbreak of genital herpes close to her due date, the following actions, taken as soon as she detects the first signs (tingling, soreness), can shorten the length of the outbreak: Remove all restrictive clothing (underwear, pantyhose, pants, etc.) so that air can circulate freely to the developing lesion. After peeing, wash and blow-dry the area gently. The goal is to get the wet lesion to crust over, after which it will heal quickly and no longer be a risk to the baby.

Make your client aware of the many benefits of staying calm and relaxed, especially in the last few weeks of her pregnancy, because herpes outbreaks are definitely linked with stress.

Trudy Noort (E-News)

For genital herpes, I suggest that immune-stimulating supplements be taken throughout pregnancy, particularly vitamin C in the mineral ascorbate form (not just ascorbic acid), plus bioflavonoids and rutin. Also try a garlic supplement. I have had great success with 5 Mushroom Extract, which is anti-viral. It contains the Japanese mushrooms *Tremella fuciform*, *Cordyseps sinensis*, *Ganoderma lucidium*, *Lentinus edodes*, *Grifola frondosa*. Take 10 to 20 drops in water three times a day.

A client of mine developed an outbreak of herpes a week before her due date; after using the extract, everything resolved in about three days.

Marianne Idle (E-News)

Prolapsed Uterus

For womb prolapses there are several good homoeopathic remedies. The most commonly prescribed are probably sepia 30c, calcium fluoride and magnesium chloride. The potency would depend on how well the remedy matched the client. The latter two can also be taken as cell salts. I'm sure some exercises could be taught by a trained physiotherapist or yoga teacher.

Glenis (E-News)

Blue Cohosh
Latin: *Caulophyllum thalictroides*
Pinyin: None
Category: Wind damp dispelling, blood quickening, stasis dispelling
Taste: Bitter, pungent
Property: Warm
Direction: Slightly dispersing

Blue cohosh has a tendency to disperse evils because it promotes sweating and dispels wind, cold and damp. It quickens the blood and moves stasis. Most blood quickeners will cause expulsion of the uterine contents because the fetus is said to be made of qi and blood. I think those women for whom blue cohosh doesn't work are those who are weak to begin with, and qi vacuity as the major cause of hemorrhage is not well served by its use. Those who may benefit from it are those who need a bit of dispersing along with moving, a pattern that may be seen in trying to initiate labor, not stop a hemorrhage.

Blue cohosh may be used for a labor tonic when there are symptoms that might indicate its use, notably blood stasis signs such as abdominal discomfort, purplish hue or spots on the tongue, rough pulse. Otherwise it seems too indirect an herb to use without cause. Due to its dispersing nature, blue cohosh may actually cause a qi vacuity, and hence, a failure of the uterus to have enough qi to accomplish normal labor.

Dosage for blue cohosh in the treatment of hemorrhage is usually 10 to 15 drops of tincture every 15 minutes, or until vomiting occurs. A decoction can be made by boiling one ounce of herb in four cups of water for 45 minutes until it is reduced to two cups. Administer one-half cup every hour.

Black Cohosh
Latin: *Cimicifuga racemosa*; Chinese species is *Cimicifuga foetida*
Pinyin: Sheng ma
Category: Wind-heat dissipating
Taste: Pungent, sweet, slightly bitter
Property: Cold
Direction: Ascending, dispersing

The functions of black cohosh are listed as upbearing yang (a form of qi), effusing exterior (wind-heat), out-thrusting papules (rashes), and resolving toxins. Upbearing yang means that black cohosh raises qi. In cases of qi vacuity where the qi sinking causes prolapse, black cohosh is absolutely indicated. Since hemorrhage can be caused by qi sinking, black cohosh should be used in the presence of prolapse. It should not be used when a retained placenta contributes to the hemorrhage, as the ascending action of black cohosh may compound the placental retention. Chinese black cohosh is not known for its antispasmodic properties (usually blood quickeners in TCM).

Black cohosh works well in tincture form. A typical dose is 15 drops every 15 minutes for acute bleeding, then 15 drops taken four times a day. Also effective for the ascending action needed for sinking qi is an infusion of one ounce to two cups of water, boiled for about seven minutes. Administer in one-half cup doses twice a day.

Cayenne
Latin: *Capsicum frutescens*
Pinyin: None
Category: Interior warming
Taste: Spicy
Property: Hot
Direction: None noted

Even though cayenne is sometimes said to be hemostatic, this action can only be applied to certain types of bleeding, such as external trauma. Midwives have reported to me that when they tried cayenne for hemorrhage the bleeding would stop for awhile, only to return about 20 minutes later with a vengeance. Interior warming herbs strongly warm the center—the source of essential qi—and thus in cases of hemorrhage from qi vacuity, may have some benefit in warming the yang and restoring the proper qi function of containing the blood. This, however, is indirect in action. The danger of using cayenne is that should there be some element of heat in the blood as a causative factor, the cayenne can greatly exacerbate the hemorrhage. I would not use it for a serious bleed, even as a "carrier" to move other herbs into the circulation, unless I was absolutely sure that warming the yang was one of the things I really wanted to do. Cayenne could conceivably be used for a person who is pale, chilled, with a watery hemorrhage, pale tongue and slow pulse, but never for anyone with heat signs. Since pregnancy confers some heat and most pregnant women experience a rise in pulse rate as part of this, I would suspect cayenne is rarely indicated for hemorrhage. Giving cayenne in the prenatal period may actually contribute to hemorrhage.

Shepherd's Purse
Latin: *Capsella bursa-pastoris*
Pinyin: ji cai
Category: Blood stanching
Taste: Pungent, sweet
Property: Cool
Direction: Contracting

Blood stanching medicinals comprise a category of herbs used for what is called "branch of root" and "branch treatment." This means that instead of treating a root cause of a disorder, the manifestation of the disorder is seen as so urgent that it is treated first. Hemorrhage is one of those situations where the emergency need of stopping bleeding becomes paramount in the treatment.

Shepherd's purse is well known in the East and West for its ability to stop bleeding. Many serious bleeds may have some element of heat in the blood, and the cooling properties of shepherd's purse may address the need to eliminate heat.

If a tincture is given, effective doses may be up to 30 ml. As an infusion, one-half ounce of dry herb infused for 15 minutes in one cup of water is effective. Do not give shepherd's purse as a preventative. In normal childbirth some bleeding should occur because it discharges "old blood" that might otherwise create problems in the postpartum period or later. To give someone a blood stanching herb in the absence of need could create problems where none existed before.

(Continued on next page)

CAUSE OF HEMORRHAGE	SIGNS and SYMPTOMS	HERBS
QI VACUITY	Profuse, watery, sometimes pale bleeding, accompanied by weakness, general lack of strength, shallow pale complexion, feeble voice, spontaneous sweating, aversion to chills, a pale tongue, and a weak, thin pulse	Chinese ginseng, cotton root bark, blue cohosh
QI SINKING	Qi vacuity signs as above, with the addition of prolapse (cervical or uterine)	Qi vacuity herbs as above with the addition of black cohosh
BLOOD STASIS	Dark red-purple to black bleeding with clots that can be small or large, fixed pain, a dull, dark facial complexion especially around the lips (not to be confused with cyanosis), a tongue that is purplish or has ecchymotic areas to it, and what is known as a rough pulse	Motherwort, pseudoginseng
HEAT	Profuse, bright red, or thick bright red bleeding accompanied by a sensation of heat, red face or red cheeks, thirst, dry mouth and tongue, irritability, dark urine, a red tongue or just red at the tip, and a rapid full or rapid fine pulse	Shepherd's purse, motherwort, cotton root bark, avoid Chinese ginseng, no cayenne

To stop bleeding in any of the above situations, either shepherd's purse or pseudoginseng can be added to the herbs that treat the pattern.

Pseudoginseng

Latin: *Panax pseudoginseng*
Pinyin: San Qi
Category: Blood stanching
Taste: Sweet, slightly bitter
Property: Warm
Direction: Ascending, dispersing

Pseudoginseng is another blood stanching herb that is used simply to stop bleeding as a branch treatment. It also has the ability to quicken the blood and dispel stasis, so it is useful in postpartum hemorrhage, especially where there is dark purple-red bleeding, clots or pain.

Pseudoginseng is available in powdered form in the Chinese patent known as Yun Nan Bai Yao (sometimes spelled Yunnan Pai Yao). It may be found in powder or encapsulated form. The powder is more rapidly assimilated and is better for use in postpartum hemorrhage. The powder is administered in water; be aware that it doesn't dissolve so it must be drunk as a sort of sludge. Use about one teaspoon per one-half cup water, taken every 15 minutes or as needed. Do not use as a preventative.

Yun Nan Bai Yao comes with a small red pill that is separate from the powder or capsules. The pill is for shock only, not for the prevention of shock. It contains aromatic herbs of the orifice-opening category that act much like smelling salts. These herbs are very dispersing and shouldn't be used unless someone has lost consciousness.

Yun Nan Bai Yao is indicated for a swollen, bruised or torn perineum unless accompanied by great debility and fatigue due to blood loss. Then it may be too moving if used alone.

Motherwort

Latin: *Leonurus cardiaca* in the West; *Leonurus heterophylli* in the East
Pinyin: Yi mu cao
Category: Blood quickening, stasis dispelling
Taste: Pungent
Property: Cool
Direction: Ascending, dispersing

Motherwort is used for hemorrhage characterized by dark purple-red bleeding, clots and/or abdominal pain. This kind of hemorrhage is due to blood stasis and unless the stasis is removed, the blood will continue to flow outside the normal channels. You must quicken the blood to stop it, and motherwort is relatively safe for this use. In Western language motherwort is a uterine stimulant, relaxant, cardiac tonic and carminative.

The dosage is one ounce of herb to four cups water, boiled down to two cups, then taken in half-cup doses as often as every 15 minutes if need be, but more likely two times a day. Its vile taste aside, motherwort is the most effective treatment for afterbirth contractions.

Chinese Ginseng (also known as Kirin Ginseng or Jilin Ginseng)

Latin: *Panax ginseng*
Pinyin: Ren shen
Category: Qi supplementing
Taste: Sweet, slightly bitter
Property: Slightly warm
Direction: Ascending

Ginseng strongly boosts qi and
(Continued on next page)

works effectively on the hemorrhage from qi vacuity and qi sinking. It is such a valuable herb that it is worth its high price to have it on hand after a birth. Since some loss of qi and blood is seen as inherent in even normal childbirth, this is the one herb that can be given without further indication. There are many types of ginseng. American and Siberian ginseng do not have the same properties.

I always boil about one-half to one ounce in two cups water for an hour or so during a labor just to have it on hand. It boils down to just a cup, so keep an eye on it when it's cooking.

Cotton Root Bark

Latin: *Gossypium herbaceum*
Pinyin: None
Category: Yang supplementing
Taste: Sweet, sour
Property: Warm
Direction: Descending

Cotton root bark works on qi vacuity because it warms and supplements yang (meaning function), especially the yang function of holding the yin (blood). It also stimulates contractions and descends the placenta. If there is one herb that is useful almost anytime someone hemorrhages, it's this one. It won't make anyone sick like blue cohosh might and is much more reliable for induction.

References

Bensky, D. & Gamble, A. (1993). *Chinese Herbal Medicine Materia Medica*, Rev. Ed. Seattle, Wash.: Eastland Press.
Flaws, B. (1993). *The Path of Pregnancy*, Vol. 1. Boulder, Colo.: Blue Poppy Press.
Ody, P. (1993). *The Complete Medicinal Herbal*. London: Dorling Kindersley.
Tierra, M. (1988). *Planetary Herbology*. Twin Lakes, Wis.: Lotus Press.
Wiseman, N. (1995). *Fundamentals of Chinese Medicine*, Rev. Ed. Brookline, Mass.: Paradigm Publications.

Chinese Patent Remedy for Hemorrhage

by Valerie Hobbs, Midwife, Doctor of Chinese Medicine

A CHINESE PATENT remedy, Yun Nan Bai Yao (also known as Yunnan Pai Yao), is made entirely of one herb whose pharmaceutical name is *Radix Pseudoginseng*, its pinyin (Chinese) name is san qi, and its Latin name is *Panax notoginseng* or *Panax pseudoginseng*. This herb is similar in morphology to Panax ginseng (or Chinese ginseng), but its properties are entirely different.

Whereas Chinese ginseng supplements "qi" (that is, it increases energy and organ function), Yun Nan Bai Yao stops bleeding. It also "quickens" what is called blood stasis. Blood-stanching (the stopping of bleeding) medicinals comprise a category of herbs used for the "branch" portion of "root-and-branch" treatment. This means that instead of treating a root cause of a disorder, the manifestation of the disorder is seen as so urgent that it is treated first. Hemorrhage is a situation where the need to stop bleeding becomes paramount in the treatment; therefore, herbs in the blood stanching category are some of the midwife's best friends. I feel that a blood stancher should always be part of the treatment of hemorrhage.

Chinese medicine considers many and varied causes of bleeding, such as abnormal heat, both vacuous and replete (meaning empty and excess). In hemorrhage, this usually results in a heavy, profuse, thick, bright red flow. Blood stasis can also cause abnormal bleeding, i.e., the blood actually blocks the normal channel of flow, so the blood flows out of the vessels much like a stream overflowing a log dam. Unless the stasis is resolved, bleeding will continue. This type of bleeding is usually characterized by a darker, "clotty" flow and is accompanied by pain.

Two other types of bleeding are caused by a "qi" vacuity; that is, the normal energy and organ function are weak. The first of these is a spleen qi vacuity. In Chinese medicine, the spleen is responsible for "holding" blood within the vessels. This type of hemorrhage is profuse, pale or watery and often occurs in a slow trickle, and the woman is typically exhausted and pale. The second type of qi vacuity hemorrhage is when the qi is "sinking." This is also a malfunction of the spleen, which is supposed to ascend energy in the body and keep things from falling or "sinking." This type of hemorrhage is the same as spleen qi vacuity hemorrhage, with the addition of prolapse or a heavy downward falling feeling in the abdomen.

Yun Nan Bai Yao has the unique quality of stopping bleeding and resolving stasis at the same time. Because a blood-stanching herb acts on the emergency symptom, it works regardless of cause, so you don't have to spend much time or brain power figuring out the difference.

Yun Nan Bai Yao comes in three forms: a powder, encapsulated powder and a hard-to-find alcohol extract. The powders come with a small red pill. The red pill is not Radix Notoginseng, so don't make the mistake of thinking it is a stronger form of the herb. The red pill is made of herbs for loss of consciousness. The herbs are very aromatic, somewhat like smelling salts, only here they are in an oral form. This red pill will greatly scatter the energy, which is something you want if someone needs treatment for loss of consciousness but not for hemorrhage itself. If the hemorrhage is from a qi vacuity and you give the red pill, you may exacerbate the condition that caused the hemorrhage by scattering already vacuous qi; you may actually precipitate shock. If you can't remember this, then remember to throw the red pills away. It's better not to use them than to use them incorrectly.

Because the capsules will take time to break down, it is advisable to use the powder for a postpartum bleed. The powder will form a suspension in water. It won't completely dissolve. Place about one teaspoon in 1/2 cup water, stir vigorously and have the woman chug the swill. You can

(Continued on next page)

give up to half the small vial in this way, but if it doesn't work within just a few minutes, go on to the next thing in my protocol, or combine the stop-bleeding treatment with something that addresses the cause of the hemorrhage.

The capsules are useful for other, less urgent bleeds, such as prolonged postpartum bleeding and to aid healing around surgery. The dose is two capsules four times a day. If you know someone is having surgery, have them take two capsules the last time they're allowed anything by mouth and the first thing after the surgery. They can then continue with the dosage above.

Yun Nan Bai Yao, as a blood mover, is contraindicated for bleeding during pregnancy. These bleeds are sometimes caused by the same etiologies as postpartum bleed, but in pregnancy it is vital to be sure of the cause before giving something that might move the blood, as blood movers may cause the fetus to abort. So don't make a mistake; differentiate! (And don't guess.)

McZand Herbals, a manufacturer of Chinese classic herbal tinctures, is introducing tinctures with a new distillation process that makes them very effective. McZand will be marketing a hemostatic formula that midwives could use as a blood stancher in treating postpartum hemorrhage of any kind. I believe this formula will be much more effective than Yun Nan Bai Yao. McZand typically sells only to people trained to use TCM formulas, so you may have to procure it through a friendly acupuncturist.

I want to address the rumor that some midwives have begun to use Yun Nan Bai Yao to prevent hemorrhage in a woman who is not having abnormal bleeding. The false reasoning that if something is good when indicated it must be just as good when not indicated is almost like using Pitocin prophylactically. Herbs are drugs. They need to be used with full understanding of how they work and should never be applied in a manner in which they are not intended.

That said, Yun Nan Bai Yao is one of the few herbs that can be used to stop bleeding with relatively few side effects. However, since it is also a blood quickener—and that means that energetically it moves the vital substance called blood in a qi vacuity (meaning lack of energy)—given prophylactically, it could theoretically cause a bleed when there isn't one. However, Yun Nan Bai Yao, being a styptic and blood mover, can be used whenever there is trauma, such as for an episiotomy or tear, even in qi vacuity, as long as there is indication for its use. That indication can be surgery, trauma or bruising, and not necessarily a postpartum bleed.

Most likely, those who might use this herb prophylactically won't see any kind of deleterious effects in the relatively small numbers of private practice. This is because the doses given are still rather small. They are large enough to be effective when indicated, but small enough not to generate unwanted side effects—most of the time. It is also the gentle nature of the particular herb that contributes to its not producing side effects.

The problem in using any blood stancher without indication is that it can potentially stop the normal flow of blood. In childbirth, you want normal bleeding to occur, as this discharges "old blood" that might otherwise create problems in postpartum or in the future. The failure to adequately discharge the old blood is one of the causes in Chinese medicine of what we would call postpartum depression and psychosis and sets up the condition of blood stasis, a cause of afterbirth pains in later pregnancies. So, to give someone a blood stanching herb in the absence of having a need to stop bleeding could create problems where none existed.

As I pointed out above, Yun Nan Bai Yao avoids this problem because it has a secondary function of quickening the blood, but it is still primarily a blood stancher. So, if you are tempted to give a blood stancher as a preventative, please avoid it. Preventatives should be basically foods or vitamins, where a known deficiency will cause a known problem. This logic is misdirected when applied to herbal medicines. Herbal substances can have a powerful effect, plus side effects, and should never be applied without knowing fully how they work and why.

Tips & Tricks

Herbs, Exercise & Nutrition

I am a student midwife and work with herbs. Two herbs helpful for diabetes and safe during pregnancy are buchu and uva ursi. The dosage would be: as a tea, boil a heaping teaspoon of uva ursi in a pint of boiling water for 30 minutes (low boil to prevent evaporation). Remove from heat and add an ounce of buchu leaves. Steep. Do not boil buchu leaves. Buchu is originally from Africa. If you have trouble finding the ingredients, I can help you.

Louise Hay states a probable cause for diabetes is "longing for what might have been; great need to control; deep sorrow; no sweetness left." The affirmation she recommends is, "This moment is filled with joy. I now choose to experience the sweetness of today." I have seen metaphysical work effect healing.

As a fitness trainer, I was taught how exercise and nutrition help diabetes. Exercise promotes the entry of glucose into the cells and so can lower a diabetic's glucose levels. Too much exercise can bring on an episode of hypoglycemia. A safe recommendation, with your care provider's approval, would be: walking, plenty of hydration and the Bradley or Brewer diet (which can be accommodated to vegetarians). One key to stabilizing blood sugar is the required 75-100 grams of protein daily, eaten in six meals throughout the day. Pasta should be cooked al dente. White flour/sugar products should be replaced with whole grains. Carbohydrates break down into sugar, so limit portions.

Beth (E-News)

Hypertension Treatment

A client alleviated her hypertension by taking two droppersful (could have taken three) of hawthorn berry tincture, one in the morning and one at night. I had also recommended supplementing with calcium/magnesium (1000-1200mgs/500-600mgs). She took these tablets in the morning and at night to get the full amount.

Constance Miles (E-News)

Homeopathic Remedies for the Midwife

by Lisa Goldstein, CPM, CNM

Through the years, as I have become more acquainted with homeopathics, I have found some that have become real lifesavers for me. They may be old friends to you, too, but perhaps you will find some new ones on this list, or new uses for old friends.

Aconite

I use this remedy most often to alleviate feelings of fear. When I have to talk to someone I don't know about something serious or important, I make sure to have aconite in my pocket. If the situation becomes tense, I excuse myself and go to the bathroom, where I take a few quick drops or pellets of the remedy, depending on what I have on hand.

Arnica

What a friend this one is! For any kind of tissue trauma, think arnica—even if the injury happened some time ago. Or, if you've studied until you feel like you have "no more" brain left, arnica helps ease brain cell trauma, too. Arnica is a good remedy, as it is one that can be used in a topical form as well. In fact, I have

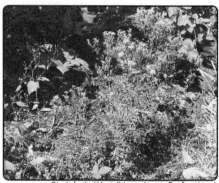
St. John's Wort (Hypericum Perforatum)

days that I wouldn't be able to move certain joints if I didn't have arnica oil rubbed on them. It is particularly useful after a long and hard labor: I like to give the mom a sponge bath, then rub down her back and legs with arnica oil. When I get home, I put a few drops of the oil in my bathtub and have a good soak before I go to sleep. I know that I won't wake up sore, and neither will the new mom.

Bryonia

There's a certain kind of right-sided headache that I sometimes get, especially if I've had to endure being in a room with a smoker. One of the characteristics to let you know you need this remedy is a grumpy (bearlike) kind of "leave me alone" mood. This remedy works well to alleviate the pain.

Carbo Veg.

My college-age sons call this one "Turbo Veg." due to its capacity to alter the state of exhaustion. When I'm at a labor that goes into Day 2 and everyone in attendance feels like zombies, I walk around the room and give each person two drops of this remedy. In a few minutes, if a person does not feel a lot better, I give two more drops. I know this remedy has literally saved my life: After taking two drops, I've been able to drive home without falling asleep at the wheel, even though I was exhausted. Another benefit of this remedy is that there are no aftereffects. When I get home, I am still able to go right to sleep.

Ferrum Phos.

I used to get a certain kind of sore throat repeatedly if I was feeling really "run down." I would feel the sore throat coming on and then I knew I was in for it. Now, when I feel the first sensations of soreness, out comes the ferrum phos. It usually works on the first dose; sometimes I need another one later, but that is usually all. I haven't been sick with a sore throat now for many years.

Gelsemium

This homeopathic is for performance anxiety. I like to combine it with aconite, as the situation warrants. I used gelsemium a lot during the first few weeks of nursing school. It really helps before a test, too, especially if you were up the previous night catching a baby instead of studying.

Glonoine

This one has several spellings; one of the others is glonoinum. I just call this remedy "heat drops" because that's what we use them for, as they act like liquid air conditioning. You probably shouldn't use them frivolously, but when you really need them, they are wonderful. I suffered from heat stroke a few years ago. Now if I get overheated, I have a very bad reaction: I heat up quickly, becoming very sick and dysfunctional. But if I take these drops, I'm usually fine. Glonoine is always in my pocket in the summer months, especially when I'm riding my bicycle.

St. John's Wort (Hypericum Perfor...)

Ignatia

This is a useful remedy for grief. If you are sighing a great deal, this remedy may be what you need. It is even useful to heal things that happened a long time ago. There are times when this one has been my lifeline—I'm very grateful to know it's there. If I am unable to get past old issues, I take ignatia before going to sleep. I often have dreams that give me particular insights that help with the problem of the moment. Also, it is a very good remedy to use after an unexpected or bad outcome. It helps to give you a better perspective on the situation, rather than becoming lost in the grief. Don't forget to leave some with the parents too.

(Continued on next page)

Hypericum

This remedy helps with pain, especially in an area that is full of nerve tissue, such as your hand. If you slam it in the car door, hypericum will stop the throbbing pain (then you don't have to admit to anyone that you did something that stupid!).

Kali Bichromicum

We call this homeopathic Kali Bi for short. This sinus remedy enabled me to stop using pseudoephedrine for my chronic sinus trouble (believe it or not, my nose has been broken 13 times). When I feel pressure building in my sinuses, Kali Bi comes to the rescue, and results for me are within minutes.

Kali Muriaticum

We call this remedy Kali Mur. It works similarly to Kali Bi, but is more specific to nasal congestion that makes you feel as if you can't breathe through your nose (such as with a bad cold or flu). Instead of reaching for the nose spray that can become addictive in just three days (really!), try using some Kali Mur. The first time I tried it, my nose cleared before I put the lid completely back on the bottle—no kidding!

Staphysagria

This remedy helps me get to the heart of a situation. If taken before bed, I often have dreams that are useful to this end, and the dreams may give me the time I need to work through to a solution. It helps you to move from your head (intellect) into what you are really feeling about a situation.

For more information: to receive a product list and information please send a long envelope SASE to: Midwifery In The Moutains, Lisa Goldstein, CPM, CNM, 823 Hannah Br. Rd., Burnsville, NC 28714

Grieving and Healing: Miscarriage

by Holly Richardson

MISCARRIAGE OCCURS IN 20 percent to 25 percent of all "acknowledged" pregnancies. It is generally accepted that the actual rate probably runs between 50 percent and 75 percent of conceptions. It is estimated that almost 1 million acknowledged pregnancies end in miscarriage each year. Seventy-five percent of these occur within the first 12 weeks.

How Can We Help Women Who Suffer Miscarriages?

- Be aware that most women grieve over a miscarriage, though some will only grieve a little, or not at all.
- Be aware that most men want information about miscarriages and about what they can do for their partner.
- Use the term miscarriage, not abortion; baby, not "products of conception," and so forth.
- In subsequent pregnancies, acknowledge that parents may fear another miscarriage.
- It may be appropriate to suggest an ultrasound to reassure parents that a subsequent pregnancy is viable.
- Recognize that many women feel guilty about a miscarriage. Please reassure them!
- Make a special effort to meet with the parents for a follow-up visit four to six weeks after the loss.
- Listen, listen, listen!
- Remember, as author Sherry Jiminez says, "What is a miscarriage, but an early stillbirth."
- Let parents know that there are resources for obtaining ways to memorialize the miscarried baby/babies, such as miniature coffins, tiny clothes and so on.

Editor's Note: See Midwifery Today Issue No. 29 to read more about grieving by this author.

This "Postpartum Depression Brew," from *Wise Woman Herbal for the Childbearing Year*, by Susun Weed, can help with the postpartum symptoms that follow miscarriage.

    1/2 oz. dried licorice root (*Glycyrrhiza glabra*)
    1 oz. dried cut raspberry leaf (*Rubus idaeus*)
    1 oz. dried cut rosemary leaves (*Rosmarinus officinalls*) for depression
    1 oz. skullcap leaf (*Scutellaria lateriflora*) for a relaxing nervine

Mix the dried herbs thoroughly. Use two teaspoons per cup of boiling water. Licorice favorably affects the hormonal balance and cheers the spirits. Raspberry leaf tones the uterus and ovaries and increases available calcium, making life seem easier.

Rosemary increases the milk flow, adds calcium, tones the liver, and is a Wise Woman favorite for depression. Skullcap is also a source of calcium and is a superb nerve strengthener and soother; prolonged use establishes emotional calm.

A Holistic Approach to "Loose Cervix"

by Anna Lipo

MISCARRIAGE HAS BECOME a path of learning for me. I lost two children to what allopathic medicine calls an "incompetent cervix." I choose to call it a "loose cervix." I decided to research loose cervices both because I have one, and because this condition receives little attention.

A loose cervix is one that will not stay closed once the baby puts a certain amount of pressure on it. It usually opens in the second trimester, allowing the baby to be born when it is still too young to survive. 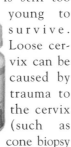 Loose cervix can be caused by trauma to the cervix (such as cone biopsy or numerous past births); by the fertility drug DES (diethylstilbestrol), which was given to many women in the 1960s and 1970s to help prevent miscarriage; or by unknown causes.

Allopathic medicine's answer to this problem is a suture around the cervix. It is like a purse string stitch holding the cervix in place. The stitch is usually put in between the 14th and 18th weeks of pregnancy. Regular visits to a doctor are required throughout the pregnancy to check the woman's cervix. By the 38th week the suture is removed. There are many accounts of women birthing their babies at home after having the suture removed!

After my first miscarriage, I was shocked to learn that one out of every five pregnancies ends in miscarriage, 80 percent occur in the first 12 weeks. As much as I had read on natural pregnancy and childbirth, I had no idea the chance of miscarriage was so high. I believed that because I was young and healthy, my pregnancy would proceed like the pictures I saw in books of women glowing and active in their last months of pregnancy—unhindered by their bulging bellies.

Looking back, I realize how little miscarriage was emphasized in the books I read. For example, *Spiritual Midwifery* has more than 100 birth stories—only one is about a woman who suffered a miscarriage. Not only does miscarriage seem under-represented in literature, it is suppressed socially as well. After I miscarried, I learned that both my aunts had miscarriages. It was never talked about until it happened to me. Our society does not allow women to grieve sufficiently after this common loss.

The holistic approach to loose cervix offered here is given either to complement the conventional medical treatment or to try on its own. I suggest doing everything possible, because it is so traumatic to lose a child.

After a miscarriage, the most important thing for the woman to do is relax so that she can heal physically and emotionally. She should allow a partner, friend or relative to take care of her. I recommend these remedies:

Drink red raspberry leaf (*Rubus idaeus*) tea (infusion) to heal and tone the uterus. It is high in many vitamins and minerals, particularly calcium, iron, phosphorus, potassium and vitamins B, C and E.

Drink nettle leaf (*Urtica dioica/urens*) tea (infusion) to help aid recovery and restore the mother's energy. Nettles also contain lots of vitamins and minerals. They are especially high in iron, calcium, vitamins A and K and chlorophyll.

The body's reaction to miscarriage is the same as to giving birth. Hormone levels change drastically. To help balance hormones and to help alleviate depression, I suggest eating figs, sprouts, royal jelly, bee pollen, ginseng and sarsaparilla. Vitex (*Vitex agnus-castus*) tincture can also be taken to balance hormone levels. I recommend trying 40 drops every morning for as long as five or six months.

For depression, the woman should take lemon balm (*Melissa officinalls*) as an infusion. I suggest one to two cups daily for one to two weeks.

Essential oil of rose can be added to a carrier oil (almond, apricot kernel, and so on) and used for massage. It is recommended when there is sadness related to the reproductive system. It can also be used in a bath, but the woman must wait at least two weeks after the birth for the cervix to close.

When the pregnancy ends in the second trimester, usually the woman's milk will come in. To dry up the milk supply, try sage leaf tea. Use two grams infused in three to four cups of water and advise the woman to drink two to four cups a day for up to two weeks.

Allow the heart to heal as well as the body. Talk about the experience if possible. It helped me a lot in working through and releasing the pain.

Burying my babies was a tremendous source of healing. I was able to say goodbye and release much of my grief. The woman might consider having a "letting go" ritual. She should find a sacred place in nature, somewhere that is special to her. After a hole is dug in the earth, she should put something into the hole that represents her loss, pain and sadness. Counsel her to visualize anything she wants to let go of flowing back into the earth. Tell her to cry, scream, whisper, sing into the hole, to visualize all this going back into the earth. Help her to breathe, let it go, bury it and leave it behind. Tell her she can always come back to this special, sacred spot.

(Continued on next page)

When the woman decides to get pregnant again there are many precautions to take with a history of late (second trimester) miscarriage. Much care needs to be taken to assure that the baby stays in the womb for the whole pregnancy. This means that all emmenogogues (substances that promote menstruation) should be avoided. Thousands of herbs are emmenogogues and contra-indicated in pregnancy (especially high risk). Learning the properties of these herbs is best for knowing what to avoid.

Emmenagogues

Bitters—some include: southernwood, wormwood, barberry, celandine, mugwort, goldenseal, rue, feverfew, tansy, sage, motherwort.

Alkaloid-containing—some include: coffee, black and green tea, barberry, goldenseal, mandrake, bloodroot.

Volatile oil-containing—some include: juniper, pennyroyal, oregano, parsley, nutmeg, ginger, rosemary, peppermint, rue, cinnamon, thuja, sage, most of the mint family.

Anthraquinone-containing—some include: senna, alder buckthorn, cascara, aloe latex.

Also avoid—spokeroot, mistletoe, cotton root, dong quai, peruvian bark.

Be aware that a dose of 6,000 milligrams of vitamin C has an emmenagogue effect.

Some common cooking herbs that may encourage miscarriage include basil, caraway, celery, saffron, tarragon, ginger, horseradish, savory, sage, thyme, marjoram, nutmeg, rosemary, parsley, watercress, oregano.

It is best to allow six to 12 months before the next pregnancy for the body to recover—and the soul, too. Both the woman and her partner should eat well, including whole grains and lots of vegetables. They should forgo smoking and reduce alcohol intake.

Certain herbs can help to prevent miscarriage, especially if the woman knows she has a loose cervix and is taking precautions on all levels. A tonic formula is used to strengthen and tone the uterus and cervix. This formula should be taken at least four months before conception at 60 drops (2 ml) three times a day. This is a general formula for a loose cervix. It may need modification depending on the woman using it:

False unicorn is a very sacred plant for women with loose cervices. It is recommended for women who have had repeated miscarriages. *King's Dispensary* says that false unicorn has the potential of "In diseases of the reproductive organs of females, esp. of the uterus…(one of four most valuable agents)…gradually removing abnormal conditions…to remove tendency to repeated and successive miscarriages…." In *American Materia Medica—Therapeutics and Pharmacognosy*, Finley Ellingwood, MD, writes that false unicorn "has a tonic influence, in general relaxation…of uterine structures. Specific in prolapsus, with a dragging or pulling down sensation in the lower abdomen." Its specific indication is strengthening to the uterus.

Cramp bark is an herb used to prepare the uterus for childbirth when there is a history of miscarriage. Its antispasmodic action acts as a uterine sedative.

Blue cohosh is used as a uterine tonic, especially with weakness or loss of tone. It has a good reputation for helping prevent miscarriage. According to *The Complete Woman's Herbal*, by Anne McIntyre, "The anti-spasmodic action helps to ensure that the uterus holds the growing baby, so it prevents premature delivery."

The loose cervix formula needs to be altered as soon as the woman decides to conceive again. Blue cohosh should be taken out of the formula. It can prevent the fertilized egg from attaching to the uterine wall. The dosage should be decreased to 10 drops three times a day once she is pregnant.

- 2 parts false unicorn
  (*Chamaelirium luteum*)
- 1 part blue cohosh
  (*Caulophyllum thalictroides*)
- 1 part cramp bark
  (*Viburnum opulus*)

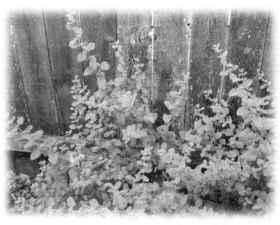

Lemon Balm

Here are additional suggestions to help your client prevent miscarriage:

600 IUs of vitamin E a day should be taken (keep at 50 IUs if the woman has high blood pressure, heart disease or diabetes).

Inverted yoga postures can also help prevent miscarriages (shoulder stands, the plow). The bow, the locust and the cobra are three yoga postures that can be practiced daily to tone the uterus. Refer to a yoga book to learn these postures.

There should be no intercourse for the pregnant woman; it may irritate the cervix and cause contractions to start. She can make love without intercourse. Tell her to be creative!

It is best to avoid cold or raw foods. They take extra energy to digest, and the body needs to devote energy to the work of holding the baby.

Keep the kidney area warm. Try having her wear a scarf around the lower waist.

Acupuncture may also help. There are specific holding points on the body that may help hold a baby. She should receive treatments as often as once a week, if possible.

During the pregnancy, especially after the first trimester, it is crucial for the mom to rest. She should not lift any heavy objects, jump around, dance or

(Continued on next page)

run. These are strict precautions. The woman should listen to her body and not push it. This is extremely difficult in this fast-paced world. However, a loose cervix tends to affect busy women.

Pay special attention to any dragging sensation in the pelvis, or any cramping or heavy weight in the uterus. If this is felt, the woman should lie down immediately. She needs a partner or friend by her side for support and someone to call her midwife and/or doctor.

All the information given is relevant to every woman dealing with a loose cervix, although the treatment she chooses should vary depending on her individual situation. To treat holistically means to focus on all dimensions of life and health—to use food, exercise, herbs, acupuncture, massage and allopathic medicine, if necessary. I hope this information may be helpful to women who have loose cervices. I wish us all a happy, healthy pregnancy and birth.

Editor's Note: *This article has been abridged from its original printed version.*

> ### Tips & Tricks
> **Carpal Tunnel Remedies**
> I have had great results in my office with an acupuncturist treating carpal tunnel in pregnancy.
> *Sara Liebling, CNM, (E-News)*
>
> I sought the help of a chiropractor for carpal tunnel syndrome with great success. Even after working in the massage business for five years, the condition has not recurred. Chiropractic adjustments, massage, stretching, reducing stress, good nutrition and adequate rest are all recommended. A drugless approach is best; the American Academy of Pediatrics committee on drugs has stated that "there is no drug either by prescription, over the counter or food additive that has ever been proven safe for the unborn baby."
> *A.T. (E-News)*
>
> Carpal tunnel seems to have become a catchall term for wrist pain. I am an exercise physiologist, so I treated my wrist pain after my son was born as an overuse injury, e.g., tendonitis. It responded well to ice (I did this while nursing), rest (especially when nursing it is important to use a nursing pillow or many pillows), and especially long-term chiropractic adjustments. Make sure that when carrying your baby you switch sides so that both wrists, arms, hips, etc., share the work. And acupuncture is extremely effective for soft tissue injuries, which this usually is.
> *Kyle Harrow (E-News)*
>
> When pregnant moms come into my store/office and mention the problem of their wrist hurting, I ask them if they want to try a magnetic wristband. They have all been very surprised when it doesn't hurt anymore within 10 to 15 minutes. But remember, magnetic therapy products are not all created equal. I only use the big name from Japan!
> *PJ Jacobsen, IBCLC (E-News)*

Herbal Protocol for Group B Strep

by Betty Idarius, LM

I HANDLE GROUP B STREPTOCOCCUS BY giving women information on it regarding the risks, treatment, etc., and leave it up to them whether to culture or not. If they choose to culture, I do it at about 35 weeks. If the culture is positive, I give them the choice of herbal protocol and reculturing in two weeks to make sure the herbs worked. Or they can take antibiotics orally when labor starts.

The herbal protocol I recommend is as follows (it works for GBS, trichomonas or chlamydia):

1. Add 1/2 teaspoon goldenseal tincture to 2 cups body temperature spring water. Add this to a douche bag and douche once a day for a week.
2. Also take 500 mg golden seal (or 1/4 tsp. tincture) orally three times a day.
3. Then, use a lactobacillus implant daily for two weeks (a gelatin capsule of high quality lactobacillus inserted vaginally once or twice a day works well).

It is important to teach women how to douche properly. Lying on a towel in the bathtub works well. She can put some pillows under her hips to elevate them. Make sure the tip of the douche is NOT inserted into the cervix. Have her undo the douche clip until the air is out of the line and reclip. As she slowly lets the fluid out, she should hold her labia closed with the fingers of one hand. This allows the vaginal tissues to expand and the fluid to wash over all the mucosa. As she holds her labia closed, her vaginal mucosa will balloon out. Some fluid will run out anyway, but keeping as much in as possible for at least a few minutes is recommended.

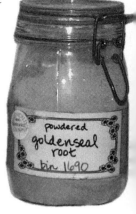

Be sure to reculture after the two weeks are up to make sure the GBS is gone. Then occasional douching, oral goldenseal tincture, and vaginal acidophilus is recommended so she doesn't recolonize. I don't have a definite routine on that.

If the pregnant woman chooses to use antibiotics, this is what was recommended to me by a University of California at Davis perinatologist: Amoxycillin 500 mg every four hours, beginning as soon as labor begins. The routine hospital protocol is IV ampicillin 2 grams, then 1 gram every four hours during labor, but I do not do IVs at home.

Prenatal

Teaching Moms About Prenatal Nutrition

by Sue LaLeike

THROUGH THE YEARS those of us who teach prenatal classes have noticed that despite so many different protocols existing from birth attendant to birth attendant, one constant is that the vast majority of obstetricians seldom discuss nutrition with moms-to-be—unless it's to suggest they are gaining too much weight. With the expanding availability of midwifery care, this is changing, but if most pregnant women are to learn anything about nourishing themselves and their babies, it appears it is probably going to be from inside our classrooms and prenatal clinics.

Keeping the attention of young women who are accustomed to fast-paced, colored, carefully choreographed and scripted television ads for food can be a challenge. People today are used to having all their senses appealed to at once. By mimicking this sense-assault trend and encouraging the active participation of parents-to-be in our lessons about nourishment, our advice, we hope, will be acted upon rather than relegated to some bored nook of our clients' brains.

Achieving this has been a recent topic of discussion on one of the Internet discussion groups in which I participate. When I put out requests for information to several groups, I noted with interest that all the responses I received were from fellow teachers of Bradley Method childbirth classes. Prenatal nutrition must be a strong interest for anyone teaching this variety of classes because it is part of the class outline for every single session of each series—quite a contrast, in terms of nutritional education, from what most women receive at the average obstetrical prenatal appointment.

On this topic in general, Sabrina Cuddy of Palo Alto, California, has some sage advice for the more nutritionally enthusiastic among us: "There is no point in telling women they must drop everything they currently eat and replace it with perfect, healthy, whole foods. Most women realize they have to eat carefully in pregnancy and will shut out what you have to say if you make them feel bad about their diet. However, if you give

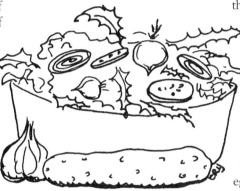

illlustration by Cynthia Yula

easy suggestions for ways to improve their diet, they will at least try."

Ask class members to maintain food diaries for at least two weeks and then give them to you for review. After reviewing the diaries, tailor what you say in class to what people actually need to hear.

In a classroom situation, have a mom-to-be describe what she feels was the healthiest meal she ate in the past week. Then using a chalk or grease board, show her how her diet adds up. Total the protein, check for overall balance, compliment her finer dietary efforts, and make any suggestions in a positive way. Alternately, draw the whole class into a similar exercise by asking them to create a fantasy meal or even a fantasy day's worth of eating that would meet a pregnant woman's nutritional needs.

I have two favorite segments that involve baskets and artificial food. The first involves teaching about fruits, vegetables and nuts. I have carefully gathered the most realistic wax fruit, plastic nuts and berries, and papier-mâché vegetables that I could find over the years. These fill a woven basket to overflowing. I pass the basket around the class and have everyone take a favorite item or two until it is empty. Then each person is asked to tell what he or she knows about the benefits of that food and how the person likes to eat it. Others can then add their comments; the classes can almost end up teaching themselves.

Another basket is filled with a dozen plastic Easter eggs, the kind that split in two for filling with treats. The basket also contains Easter grass, one of those fuzzy chicks that cheeps when held in the hand and a crocheted mama hen. In the eggs are slips of paper telling the benefits of eating eggs, as well as ways to prepare them. (This part of the activity was developed by a Bradley Method teacher; but with a little research, anyone should be able to print up their own slips of paper.) Students take out an egg or two as the basket is passed and share aloud, fortune-cookie style, what the slips say. I have also added an extra egg filled with one of those molded plastic fetal models, of about 14 weeks' gestational age. This gives the exercise a little extra impact, as well as being an appropriate activity for an early pregnancy class.

Ann Sterling, an educator from Ann Arbor, Michigan, also has some special ways to involve her couples in teaching and sharing about nutrition. In one class she has each person draw from a bowl a paper that specifies a "research assignment." The topics might include greens, water, calcium, caffeine and so forth. The person is assigned to find out about these subjects and share what he or she finds with the rest of the class a few weeks hence. For instance, what is it? Where can you get it? What does it do? Is it

(Continued on next page)

Tips & Tricks

Nausea

I suffered with nausea during my pregnancies and for years after pregnancies two and three. My internist finally diagnosed my gall bladder as the source. He said my having been pregnant was the biggest risk factor. Instead of having my gall bladder removed, I changed my diet. I reduced fat and protein, especially eliminating eggs. I added apples. I had to be very strict at first. Years later, I can eat more normally without nausea. I know some who have had the gall bladder out and it did not correct the nausea. Digestive enzymes and extracts were a help to me, but I don't know about their safety during pregnancy.

Pam Easterday (E-News)

Add Fish to Mom's Diet

By adding cold water marine fish to their diets, pregnant women and nursing mothers will be giving their babies important fats that facilitate the growth of brain and nerve cells in the developing fetus and nursing infants, according to a study at the University of Connecticut. Neither developing fetuses nor nursing infants can produce sufficient amounts of an important fatty acid, DHA (docahexanoic), on their own. Cold water marine fish include salmon, herring, tuna, swordfish, mackerel, sardines and trout.

Women's Health Weekly, 9/14/98

Boost for Placentas

Researchers at the University of Tennessee and other centers found that higher intakes of the antioxidant vitamins E, C and beta-carotene could be linked to less calcification of placental tissue caused by smoking.

The researchers suggest that a diet rich in antioxidants may also be important for pregnant nonsmokers whose placentas may be at increased risk of damage due to pregnancy-induced high blood pressure or exposure to environmental pollutants.

American Journal of Epidemiology 147, 1998, reported in Midwifery Matters, Summer 1998

good, bad, hard to get enough of, being preached against in the media? No term papers here, just incentive to do a little learning and then share with their classmates, for at least one minute and no more than five minutes, what they find out.

Ann asks her class members to bring in recipes that focus on whatever area(s) they, as a group, seem to have a hard time with. These get added to her ongoing collection from other classes, and everyone gets a copy. Common subjects have been green vegetables, brown-bag meals, and quick (or party) snacks. An added benefit for Ann is that she's ended up with quite a few new recipes that she likes to use in her own meal planning.

One idea was shared secondhand by Renee Kendall of Edmond, Oklahoma. It came to her via still another Bradley educator, Becky Hanson from Rolla, North Dakota. This one requires an easygoing coach with a sense of humor, but it certainly leaves a lasting impression on anyone who witnesses it. The procedure is to ask one of the fathers for his wallet, assuring him you will give it back. Remove all the currency in the wallet and return the wallet to him. He will now become quite uncomfortable. You say, "Oh, I'm sorry, did you want the money back, too?"

Next, hand him only part of the cash you took, saying, "Now I have enriched you!" Of course, you eventually return all the money. Now explain that when a package of food in the grocery store has a label that says "enriched," what the manufacturer has actually done is take out all the good natural nutrients and then put back some (but not all) of them. However, since they can't get all the nutrients to go back in quite the same way they occurred naturally, the manufacturer "enriches" the food by adding extra vitamins and minerals that were chemically created in a laboratory. So, just because it says new and improved, or enriched, it doesn't necessarily mean it has better food value than the food had in its original, fresh state.

Many of us provide snacks, and sometimes couples are asked to volunteer to bring things to eat during class. Some teachers ask couples to put what they've learned into action by bringing healthy snacks, or they assign a focus area, such as orange and yellow fruits and vegetables. Others take potluck. Sharing food together adds a special element to classes, whether it is a quick bite or a potluck dinner to finish out the class.

Adaptations of many of these ideas are possible in clinic situations. With the diet diaries, it is possible to offer expanded, in-depth counseling. The decor of waiting areas can be enhanced with baskets of edibles (real or artificial), and lovely prints of exotic fruits are widely available. Recipe collections could become a standard handout for some services—if not wide-ranging collections for cooking all foods, then perhaps small booklets focusing on the specific areas clients most need to incorporate into their diets. Access to a lending library of cookbooks and other nutritional information is appreciated by many moms.

I have often been asked by people if it is more important to teach a mom-to-be, or to put that funding into feeding her. Of course, the food she ingests is far more important than any other thing she does in pregnancy, if we are serious about encouraging healthy future generations. The best of both worlds is to teach pregnant women what will most safeguard her and her baby's health and well-being—how to wisely choose which foods she eats now and later, while nursing, as well as what to feed the child as it weans. Given the motivation of almost all pregnant women to eat the best they possibly can, this is a time of rich opportunity for all concerned.

illustration by Cynthia Yula

What Can Midwives Do?

by Tom Brewer, MD

WHEN A WOMAN comes under your care, assume she's undernourished. The majority of women have no idea that diet is important, even today. And if a woman comes to you late into her pregnancy and you haven't seen her before, it is never too late to get her started on the nutrition program to prevent toxemia. Never.

Tell your women to learn to graze. Small, frequent feedings is a fine way to increase dietary volume and value. Tell them not to pass the fridge or the fruit bowl without having a glass of milk, just one more egg, a small sandwich, an apple.

The only guideline I ever gave was: "Eat according to your appetite (good foods), salt to taste, drink to thirst (I caution against drinking too much water), be active and exercise, and rest when you're tired." The woman should be led to follow her own instincts. Prenatal care is what you do for yourself between visits.

Every aspect of labor is easier if the woman's diet was good during her pregnancy. Women who eat conscientiously and train to become "birth athletes" do not exhibit a lot of pain during delivery, and they find breastfeeding far easier as well.

Tell women if they eat enough calories, the protein goes to the baby and to the breast, where it belongs.

You can turn toxemia around! The status quo teaches, "Deliver the baby." Some midwives don't know what to do, and they panic. Some try to cleanse the liver with herbal remedies. But the herbal treatments have become medicalized. It's not like midwives of old who would go into the fields and forests and find their own herbs.

I threw away the things I was trained to do. Midwives will have to unlearn so much, too. The RNs who are coming into the alternative network are unlearning their medicalization. I had to unlearn also, and go back to basics, go back to nature, and let this body, this woman, this pregnancy, grow on its own steam.

Remember, if you're getting your training among wolves, you're going to act like a wolf.

The Dance of Childbirth

by Abigail Connelly

MY GREATEST ENCOURAGEMENT for a woman pregnant with life is to find celebration in her body. As women, we often celebrate our bodies with men, an amazing experience, but it would benefit our spirits so much to find this pleasure purely in ourselves as well. Dance has illuminated this pleasure for me more than any other aspect of my life.

Dance can take on many forms, or be formless. Slow movements of patience and inwardness and ecstatic outward reflections of a drumbeat all have their places in the unwinding of our souls. As Americans, it is beneficial for us to learn from other cultures. Africans teach us grounding, gather-your-power-from-the-earth movements. The women dance freely, using arms, heads and well-bent knees for expression and stability. Middle Eastern dance, also known as belly dancing, has its roots in childbirth preparation. When practiced regularly, it strengthens a woman's abdominal muscles while allowing relaxation. As a dance form it glorifies the roundness of breast and belly and enables women to experience full sensuality without its being directly related to partner sex.

Movement such as dance, with no rules or endurance tests, enables the mother-to-be to ride the currents of her energy and appreciate her body for the strong, life-giving form that it is. The exercise dance provides is good preparation for the birth itself because it promotes endurance, focus and flexibility. While dancing, one learns the value of a full breath.

More than anything, dance is a magic that lets us move with our hearts. It provides a doorway to the timeless space where we commune with all the women of the world, our mothers, grandmothers, sisters and daughters.

Thoughts on Dance

- I encourage freestyle African and belly dancing because they respect the natural positions of the body; there's no need to move it into unnatural shapes.
- If choosing a class, ask yourself: are healthy, female bodies valued; are different sizes and shapes appreciated?
- Progress at your own comfort level. Stretch before and after class. Accompany stretching with full breathing and nurturing thoughts.
- Dance groups can provide sisterly support.
- Use dance as an opportunity to adorn yourself, or to celebrate your bare belly.
- Dancing for your mate is a creative way to share yourself.
- Prenatal yoga is a very good thing. Your baby will love the joy brought by music and dance, as well as by the tranquility of yoga; and your baby's happiness will help you to feel what is truly important.
- A great joy comes from dancing outside in nature. Bare feet on the earth are a channel for the Mother's blessing.
- Dance is limitless. So are we!

Dance is an amazing medium to heal ourselves and generate energy toward our future.

illustration by Kiki Metzler

Tips & Tricks

Gestational Diabetes

With my first pregnancy I had symptoms of gestational diabetes in my last five weeks of pregnancy. I was placed on a diabetic diet and monitored my blood sugar levels at home. I found the diet strange and difficult, but followed it. I gained 35 pounds on my 5-foot-1-inch frame and did not exercise. My son was born 11 days early after a drugged labor, weighed 7 pounds, 4 ounces, and had multiple health problems. He was recently diagnosed with learning disabilities and attention-deficit hyperactivity disorder (ADHD).

During my next full-term pregnancy I followed the Brewer diet, ate a well-balanced and varied diet, and exercised regularly. I gained exactly the same amount of weight and was regularly tested for gestational diabetes, but all tests were within normal limits. I remained very healthy. My second son was born exactly on his due date after a natural labor, weighed 8 pounds, 14 ounces, was extremely healthy, and continues to be so. The only difference between the two pregnancies was diet, exercise, a midwife and education.

Amy V. Haas, AAHCC, NY

Alfalfa & Cigarettes

If the woman is a cigarette smoker, have her take 10 to 12 tablets of alfalfa a day prophylactically. This is also an effective treatment for heartburn.

Ina May Gaskin, TN

Colorful Meals

A midwife friend says she tells her clients to always make sure their food is colorful! Breakfast, lunch and dinner should be colorful and as close to its original form as possible. This way, by having yellow, red, orange and green foods on your plate, it is likely mom is eating the right things for growing a healthy baby.

Sue LaLeike, FL

Alfalfa for Good Nutrition

Alfalfa tablets are an excellent source of micronutrients and help a woman who is not getting routine good nutrition.

Tricks of the Trade Circle, NY '97

Land Food, Sea Food, Brain Food

by Michel Odent, MD

HUMAN NUTRITION includes two issues: what we eat (large meals, small snacks) and how we eat it (among familiar people, among strangers, while watching TV, or while reading *Midwifery Today* or the *Wall Street Journal*).

We will focus on what we eat

According to geneticists, we are special chimpanzees whose brain is four times bigger than the brain of our close relatives. At birth the volume of the human brain is already 25 percent of what it will be in adulthood, after a growth spurt that begins at mid-gestation. Therefore, common sense dictates that, during the second half of pregnancy, the specific needs of the developing brain should be a priority among humans. Our common sense is not in contradiction with the most recent scientific data. Where nutritional needs are concerned, it seems necessary to distinguish early pregnancy and late pregnancy.

Early Pregnancy

A recent "prospective observational study" at Princess Anne Maternity Unit, in Southampton, has assessed the average frequency of consumption of 100 foods or food groups among 655 women at different stages of pregnancy. Mothers who had high carbohydrate intakes in early pregnancy had babies with lower placental and birth weights. Although our main interest is human pregnancy, it is worth mentioning recent experiments in sheep, which have shown that high nutrient intakes in early pregnancy may suppress placental growth, resulting in reduced placental and fetal size. Such data suggest new interpretations to the commonly impaired digestive tolerance in early pregnancy, which might be seen first as an adaptive phenomenon.

A Shift in Emphasis

During the phase of rapid brain growth—i.e., the second half of pregnancy—the priority is given to a basic question: which nutrient is essential for brain development? In 1996, the answer to such a question is simple. The developing brain—which is mostly made of fat—has a thirst for one particular molecule, commonly called DHA. All midwives should know about this molecule, which is a long chain polyunsaturated fatty acid of the omega 3 family. During the last trimester of fetal life, more than 50 percent of the fatty acids that incorporate the brain are represented by DHA. I anticipate a complementary question and underline that DHA is preformed and abundant in the sea food chain (and human milk). Of course the developing brain also needs polyunsaturates from the other family (omega 6), and in particular a long chain molecule commonly called AA. These fatty acids are abundant in the land food chain, and AA is preformed and abundant in any animal food. Omega 3 and omega 6 are not interconvertible in the human body.

Until recently most research about nutrition during pregnancy has been based on protein and calorie intakes. Today our understanding of brain development as a priority offers reasons to evaluate the effects of prenatal nutritional counseling programs focusing on the balance between different families of lipids. There are other reasons for a shift in emphasis. One is that the production of the different prostaglandins involved in the regulation of the uteroplacental blood flow and the birth process are influenced by the dietary intakes of lipids. Another reason is that transfatty acids

(Continued on next page)

cross the human placenta with potential adverse effects on fetal growth. Let us recall that transfatty acids are man-made molecules whose shape is almost unknown in nature. They are abundant in such foods as processed oils, conventional margarine, cookies, french fries, fast foods, etc.

The Whipps Cross London Hospital Study

Between January 1991 and December 1992, in an east London hospital, I interviewed, at random, 499 pregnant women. This interview was offered in addition to their routine prenatal care before 20 weeks' gestation. The interview was conversational in tone and gave an opportunity to focus on the issues of brain development and transfatty acids.

In other words, women were encouraged to eat oily sea fish and to reduce their intake of foods rich in transfatty acids. To answer common questions about pollution, the coastal food chain was contrasted with the high-seas food chain. For each interviewed woman a parity matched control was established. The data regarding the perinatal period have been recently published. The mean birth weight was higher in the study group, and the difference persisted after adjusting for gestational age (85grams/ week vs. 83grams /week). The mean neonatal head circumference was greater in the study group (neonatal head circumference is a marker of brain development). The rate of delivery before 37 weeks was lower in the study group (7.3 percent vs. 9.5 percent). There were no very low weight babies (below 1500 grams) in the study group versus four in the control group. In the study group there was no eclampsia and no severe preeclamptic toxemia mentioned as "Pet" on the birth register, while in the control group, there was one eclampsia with convulsions and two severe preeclamptic toxemias.

A Mysterious Human Disease

Of course, where preeclampsia and eclampsia are concerned, statistical significance cannot be attained with a study of this dimension. We are unable to present our data alongside other similar studies because other similar studies do not exist. However, we are able to establish links with several controlled trials of the effects of fish oil supplementation during pregnancy (although eating fish should not be confused with taking capsules). Our research also reflects statistics associated with the comparatively low rate of preeclampsia in countries where the diet is rich in sea fish. My theoretical vision of human preeclampsia also takes into consideration the studies of fatty acid profiles of red blood cells—which mirrors the dietary fat intake over a two to three week period. According to M. A. Williams, women with the lowest levels of omega 3 are 7.6 times more likely to be preeclamptic than those with the highest levels.

I propose a hierarchy among the numerous biological imbalances associated with preeclampsia. The central imbalance, in my view, is the enormous discrepancy between the blood levels of DHA (the molecule essential for brain development) and the other polyunsaturates. In preeclampsia, the level of DHA remains stable. It does not drop dramatically like the level of other polyunsaturates. The price is an imbalance inside the family of omega 3 fatty acids and finally in the whole system of prostaglandins (I would need pages to enter into all the details). Such data suggest that brain development is a priority among humans: Whatever the circumstances, the levels of one of the most important molecules for brain development remain stable.

In order to simplify very complex phenomena, I propose to distinguish two critical phases in the genesis of preeclampsia. The first phase is in relation to the response of the maternal immune system at the time of placental implantation (this is confirmed by the fact that a previous miscarriage, a previous blood transfusion, or a long sexual cohabitation before conception reduces the risks of preeclampsia). The second phase—the one that is influenced by nutrition—

(Continued on next page)

Tips & Tricks

Look for Clues
A clue to whether or not a birthing woman is likely to tear is if she has noticeable stretch marks during pregnancy. Make sure she gets plenty of vitamin C with bioflavanoids (250 mg, three to four times a day).

Tricks of the Trade Circle, NY '97

Snoop a Little
What you find by looking in a woman's cupboards and refrigerator tells you much more than her diet sheet.

Lynn Baptisti Richards, AZ

Scare Tactics
One of the tricks I use in childbirth class discussion is admitting that I, too, am a junk food junkie. I tell the class that I now put more stock in the importance of nutrition than I used to. I had problems—preeclampsia, pre-term labor, horrible headaches—in all four of my pregnancies, and they can all be blamed on poor nutrition.

I tell my students that my doctors didn't know what caused me to have preterm labor which led to delivery at 36 weeks and 32 weeks, but since I didn't have good nutrition, I will always blame myself for not doing everything possible to ensure my babies' health.

Teaching by scaring? I don't know, but my students say they improve their nutrition after this class.

Suzanne Powell, CBE, GA

A Good Start
Get young women off to a good start; show each her cervix, for example, and explain what it will look like after birth. Bring them gently to self-knowledge.

Tricks of the Trade Circle, FL 1997

Circumcision
When I talk about circumcision in my childbirth classes I start out by saying we will be talking about male circumcision, although in other countries it is females who are circumcised. Many people are quite shocked and disgusted to hear there is such a thing as female circumcisions. I ask them why are they shocked? Male circumcision is medically unnecessary, and many are done in the United States.

D.B. (E-News)

Tips & Tricks

Posterior Baby and Water

If you have access to a swimming pool, float the woman belly down, for hours, if possible, with the help of a flotation device. Follow with one hour of walking. Repeat this every day for several days. The baby should turn and the mother can deliver easily.

Tricks of the Trade Circle, NY '97

Mexican Technique to Turn Baby

In Mexico, when a woman has a posterior baby, the midwife asks the woman to lie on her back on the floor, very relaxed. A rebozo (shawl) is under her lower back and hips. A midwife on each side grasps the ends of the rebozo and begins to rock the woman. The rocking motion relaxes the mom. One of the midwives suddenly pulls a little harder on her end of the rebozo, one or more times, as needed. The sudden jerk rotates the baby so its back is anterior. If you want to visualize this technique, fill a gallon jar with water and place an oversized zucchini or other squash in the jar; mark an "X" on one side of the squash. Put the lid on the jar. Lay the jar on the rebozo. With both hands, rock the jar rhythmically, then suddenly jerk on one end of the rebozo, one or more times. You'll see the squash turn over.

Tricks of the Trade Circle, NY '97

Belly Wrap to Keep Fetus Veritical

About the only time you will see a healthy grand multip at risk is if she has overstretched uterine muscles ("pendulous abdomen"). This will keep the baby from engaging, resulting in the danger of uterine prolapse, back pain and lack of progress because the baby isn't engaged or aimed at the exit. Use a "prenatal cradle" during pregnancy and have the mother labor lying down or with a "belly wrap" to help the baby stay vertical.

Rahima Baldwin Dancy, CPM

---

occurs later in pregnancy, when the fetal brain development is the most rapid and the demand in specific nutrients, and in particular long chain fatty acids, is maximum. Then the onset of a vicious cycle is possible, that is to say the disease preeclampsia. Preeclampsia appears as the price some human beings must pay for having a large brain while the nutritional supplies are not appropriate.

How We Might Prevent Preeclampsia

Not only can we propose a hierarchy among well-documented biological imbalances, but we can also establish links between different ways to reduce the risks of preeclampsia/eclampsia: the most direct way is to consume oily sea fish. This is in agreement with geographical variations in the rates of preclampsias.

For those who do not have access to the sea food chain (or who do not eat fish for individual or cultural reasons), a great importance must be given to catalysts of the metabolism of unsaturated fatty acids: only the precursor of the long chain omega 3 polyunsaturates (alpha linolenic acid) is provided by the plants of the land food chain. Magnesium is one of these catalysts, and where preeclampsia is concerned, the preventive and curative effects of magnesium are well known. Calcium is another one, and many studies have evaluated its preventive effects. Tom Brewer recalled that the Frenchman Pinard (the one who designed the fetal stethoscope) had already demonstrated, a century ago, that a milk diet could reduce the risk of eclampsia. Zinc is also a well-known catalyst of fatty acid desaturation, and preeclampsia is associated with low zinc concentration. There are many ways to provide these catalysts through the land food chain. It is worth mentioning that sea fish represents an abundant source for all of them.

It also makes sense, in order to prevent preeclampsia, to reduce as much as possible the level of blocking agents of the metabolic pathway of unsaturated fatty acids. Among them are the transfatty acids. It is significant that, according to M. A. Williams, the risk of preeclampsia is correlated with the levels of transfatty acids in the maternal red blood cells. Alcohol and pure sugar are also blocking agents of the reactions of desaturation and should be theoretically avoided; hormones such as cortisol are also known blocking agents: situations of "helplessness" (high level of cortisol) can increase the risks of preeclampsia. From a biochemical perspective, one might claim that to be happy or to eat sardines is the same—the point is to provide long chain polyunsaturates.

It is also theoretically important to avoid a fast destruction of long chain fatty acids available. That is why, during pregnancy, there is an increased need for antioxidant substances such as vitamin E, carotenoids, vitamin C and selenium. It is significant that in the regions where the soil is deprived of selenium (e.g., the Heilongjiang province in China) the rates of preeclampsia are exceptionally high. Let us underline that sea fish is also rich in selenium.

Landfood... Seafood...

It seems theoretically easier to meet the enormous needs of the developing human brain when the diet includes some food from the sea. Our focus has been on the molecules of fatty acids, which are preformed and abundant in the sea food chain. Sea foods have other characteristics, such as being rich in iodine. Iodine is also essential for brain

(Continued on next page)

development, as a major component of thyroid hormones. The imbalances between different thyroid hormones in preeclampsia also suggest that brain development is a priority among humans. Of course, the nutrients abundant in the sea food chain include salt. There is an increased need of salt during pregnancy. A sufficient amount of salt tends to moderate the stimulation of the reninangiotensin system and is also necessary for the adaptive blood dilution in late pregnancy (a sufficient amount of good quality proteins is necessary for the same reasons).

Finally, it appears that pregnant women ideally need a certain balance between food from the land and food from the sea. In the scientific context of the 1980s, one can even claim that human beings in general need such a balance. Glance through recent medical journals and you will find an impressive list of health conditions that are improved by fish oils. I mention at random: coronary heart disease, asthma, dyslexia, ulcerative colitis, Crohn's disease, eclampsia, migraines, adaptation to darkness, dysmenorrhea, attention deficit disorders, viral diseases, post viral fatigue syndrome, diabetes, multiple sclerosis, psoriasis, schizophrenia, certain cancers, rheumatoid arthritis, auto-immune nephritis and allografts intolerance.

Such a long list, plus our considerations about nutrition during pregnancy and brain development, suggest that Homo sapiens has probably been adapted to the coast at a certain phase of the evolutionary process. We should not forget that "Lucy's" bones were found eroding from the sand, lying among crab claws and crocodile eggs!

References

Godfrey, K., Robinson, S., et al. (1996). Maternal nutrition in early and late pregnancy in relation to placental and fetal growth. *BMJ* 312: 4104.
Koletzko, B. (1992). Transfatty acids may impair biosynthesis of long chain polysaturates and growth in man. *Acta Paediatr* 81: 302-6.
Lu, B., et al. (1990). Changes in selenium in patients with pregnancy induced hypertension. *Chinese J Obstet/Gynecol* 25: 325-27.
Morgan, E. (1982). *The Aquatic Ape.* London: Souvenir Press.
Odent, M., McMillan, L., Kimmel, T. (1996). Prenatal care and sea fish. *Eur J Obstet/Gynecol* 68: 49-51.
Odent, M. (1995). The primary human disease: An evolutionary perspective. *Revision* 18(2): 19-21.
Owens, J. A., et al. (1988). The effect of experimental manipulation of placental growth and development. *Fetal and Neonatal Growth.* Chichester: Wiley, 49-77.
Salvig, J. D., Olsen, S. J., Secher, J. J. (1996). Effects of fish oil supplementation in late pregnancy on blood pressure: A randomised controlled trial. *Brit J Obstet/Gynecol* 103: 529-33.
Wang, Y. K., et al. (1991). Decreased levels of polyunsaturated fatty acids in preeclampsia. *Am J Obstet/Gynecol* 164: 812-8.
Williams, M. A., et al. (1995). Omega-3 fatty acids in maternal erythrocytes and risk of preeclampsia. *Epidemiology* 6: 232-37.
Williams, M.A. (1995, Jan.). Risk of preeclampsia in relation to elaidic acid (transfatty acids) in maternal erythrocytes. S.P.O. abstracts. *Am J Obstet/Gynecol* 436: 380.

Holistically Meeting the Challenge of Infection

by Judy Edmunds, CPM, LDEM, LAM, RNC, CH

PERINATAL INFECTION CAN threaten both mother and baby. The most effective approach a midwife should take will strive for prevention and foster radiant health, which increases overall resistance to disease. Even if Plan A fails, you can be ahead of the game in correcting the situation. Start encouraging these basic habits, which, though simple, may be new to your clients:

Abundant pure water provides a medium for removal of metabolic waste. Encourage moms to drink prior to and beyond thirst. Suggest purified sources, and keep a full pitcher of water, with slices of citrus fruit or mint sprigs, chilled in the fridge. Bring water when traveling.

Regular fresh-air exercise keeps tissues oxygenated and circulates immunological factors throughout the body. Plus it decreases anxiety, increases energy and elevates mood. (Positive emotions are emerging as one of our most powerful infection fighters.)

Consistent intake of fresh, minimally processed food, including fiber and ample protein in an easily digested form, is imperative. (Delayed intestinal transit time, reduced stomach acids and diluted enzymes make items such as red meat a tough proposition.) I emphasize fresh vegetables, whole grains, plant and sea-based proteins, then fruit, in that order. Revisit this at each prenatal. Be thorough and specific in your discussion. You will be amazed to learn what some people consider a wholesome diet.

Top-quality supplements with plenty of vitamin C, bioflavonoid and minerals are a must. My favorites, in order, are: Priority One Prenatal, NF Formula's Prenatal Forte, Nutri-Natal products, and Eclectic Institute formulas. Ask at each visit how she is doing with her supplements. Can she swallow them? When does she take them? How many is she taking? Are they staying down? Suggest taking in the evening, never on an empty stomach, followed by a few bites of food. I keep a variety of formulas on hand so that we can find something agreeable that will be taken consistently. If she cannot tolerate the full amount, we come as close as possible, switching formulas as needed. Liquid supplements may temporarily get her past the queasy time. Remember protein powder if vomiting is a problem.

Intervene early—before a minor infection turns ugly. This requires careful surveillance. Allow plenty of time for prenatal visits. Pay close attention. Get all the details if something doesn't seem right. Fresh, detailed urinalysis strips, like SG 10s, give you more pieces of the puzzle, help catch things early and monitor progress.

Despite your best efforts, you will occasionally encounter infection. Now what?

(Continued on next page)

A Few of My Favorite Tools

Echinacea root and seeds (*Angustifolia, purpurea, pallida.*) Each species has slightly different actions. Blends are great, weighted in favor of angustifolia. I use this carefully studied and very safe herb prophylactically if there has been some exposure, liberally at the first sign of any infection, and throughout the healing process. Rather than just attacking the invader, it stimulates and bolsters the immune system. Many fine commercial products are available in liquid, capsule, tablets or tea.

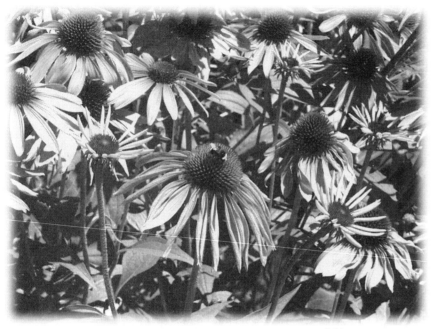

Echinacea

Fresh garlic. Acting against germs, viruses and fungi, it's inexpensive, easily obtained and harmless. (Well, yes, it smells. You can't have everything!) Used as a vaginal suppository, a peeled clove helps fight many types of infections, including yeast and bacteriosis. Chopped and added to pre-heated broth, it does a number on colds and flu. Crushed and rubbed on lacerations, it prevents sepsis. An all-around winner.

Wood-based mushrooms. I just knew there had to be some medicinal qualities to all those mushrooms I've been picking down through the years! For example, shitake (*Lentinula edodes*) is readily available and tastes wonderful. It can be generously incorporated into meals on a regular basis, or extracts can be taken as a supplement. Studies reveal shitake's immuno-potentiating and antiviral effects, its usefulness against bacterial and parasitic infections, and beneficial effects on heart and liver function.

Berberine alkaloids, found in roots of oregon grape (*Berberis aquifolium*), barberry (*Berberis vulgaris*), and goldenseal (*Hydrastis canadensis*). These bitter roots are famous for their anti-infective qualities, helping fight bacteria and yeast, and stimulating the immune system against viruses as well. Caution: these are very powerful botanicals! Internal use during pregnancy requires discernment and should be monitored by a knowledgeable practitioner cognizant of potential negative effects and educated in responsible use. Use the minimum required dose over no more than a few days. Large doses or prolonged use may cause miscarriage or liver impairment. Nevertheless, when used properly, and if needed, results can be spectacular. I like combinations with adjuvants such as peppermint, cayenne and ginger, and/or an antiseptic such as myrrh. You needn't be so circumspect with external use, as in a perineal/vulval wash. Especially if you suspect fecal matter may have contaminated vaginal lacerations or a perineal tear, consider flushing the area with strained berberine/myrrh-based tea.

Caprylic acid. If yeast has colonized a woman's "underparts," try caprylic acid internally with rosemary, thyme, pau d'arco, and plenty of acidophilus-based intestinal flora supplements to combat yeast. Externally, bathe daily, dry carefully, increase exposure of skin folds to air circulation, and apply vinegar and diluted tea tree oil to affected areas. Consider using homeopathic candida. Eliminate sugars, increase protein and chlorophyll, and don't scratch! If itching becomes unbearable, apply ice until numb. Soft cloths may be dipped in berberine-based tea and frozen for this use. (Note: protect sheets with an old towel—the roots' chartreuse pigments will stain.)

A Few Specifics

Cranberry for bladder infections, nettle for kidney, dandelion root and milk thistle for liver problems, and calendula for routine lacerations/abrasions. Consult with allied professionals for SMs, strep and staph. (Except for dire situations, I avoid antibiotics whenever possible and consider them a last resort; but, when you absolutely must use them, follow directions carefully, using the entire course, continue natural supportive remedies, and prepare to combat yeast overgrowth.)

Most infections are preventable with good hygiene and physical conditioning. When needed, nutrition and botanicals stand ready to aid restoration to health. Childbirth professionals willing to learn and apply these methods will be amply rewarded.

Calendars, Clocks and Choices

by Valerie El Halta

WHEN THE PARENTS anxiously ask, "When will our baby be born?" I usually quip: "On its birthday!" Although this answer usually elicits a giggle, it raises another question: When do we become concerned if the baby has not arrived at or around its expected dates?

We need to remember that the "expected date of delivery" is only an estimate of probable term gestation. Calculating the expected date of delivery by the last menstrual period (LMP) may be of limited validity due to many factors. Many mothers are still nursing a previous infant and have not commenced regular menses when they suspect another pregnancy. Some women have recently discontinued the use of birth control pills or injections of Depo Provera, also causing unreliable landmarks for the purposes of dating conception. All calculations are based upon a 28-day cycle, which may be widely variable. The woman with a regular 34-day cycle will ovulate later and come to term at a later date. This baby might just need to gestate a little longer.

There might also be a social reason for the mother's misreporting her LMP. Recently, a woman came to me for care very late in her pregnancy, as she had just arrived from Tijuana, Mexico. She kept saying her baby was due in another month. However, I told my friend Sol, who assisted me with translating, that she would surely deliver by the weekend. We were not surprised when she went into labor the next day.

As the baby (all 10 pounds of him) was about to be born, the mother began crying and said: "I am very worried because the baby is so premature!" As Sol translated this concern to me, I said, "I think that it is very important that this baby be early." We reassured the mom and dad that although the baby was probably quite early, he was fat and healthy and that all would be well with him.

"He is about, what? Four weeks early?" the mother asked, weeping with joy as she held her beautiful newborn baby. I later discovered that the mom was in Tijuana when she became pregnant, while the dad was in Santa Ana, California.

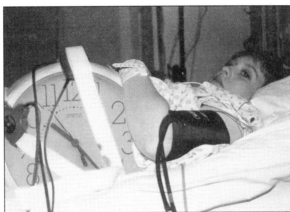

After taking all of these factors into consideration, and carefully reassessing the possible due date, it is important that we also differentiate between postdates and postterm. As I have discussed, many factors may affect date discrepancy, but it is necessary to keep in mind there is also a very real postterm syndrome.

Recent studies have concluded that true postterm babies have a higher morbidity and mortality rate, and they may be at greater risk than moderately preterm babies. Postterm syndrome appears with the following indicators: reduced placental function, reduction of amniotic fluid, non-moldability of fetal skull (resulting in hyper molding, caput formation and cephalohematoma). The woman is at greater risk for abruptio placenta, hypoglycemia and hypocalcemia, and hypoxia in labor. There is increased incidence of cephalopelvic disproportion (CPD), which may result in instrumental delivery or cesarean section, shoulder dystocia, clavicle injuries and brachial palsy. There is a much higher incidence of meconium staining, premature aspiration of meconium (in utero), meconium aspiration syndrome and more reports of "failure to thrive" babies.

Murray Enkin, et al., in *A Guide to Effective Care in Pregnancy and Childbirth*, writes, "Perinatal mortality is increased in postterm pregnancy. Prolonged pregnancy is associated with an increased risk of intrapartum and neonatal death but not of antepartum death. The risk increases with the onset of labor. A high prevalence of meconium-stained amniotic fluid is an outstanding feature among the intrapartum and asphyxial neonatal deaths. The incidence of neonatal seizures, a marker of perinatal asphyxia, is between two and five times greater in infants born after 41 weeks."

It is important, therefore, that the midwife make as accurate an estimation of gestational age as possible in order to make appropriate care choices. If the expectant mother is very unsure of her dates, for whatever reason, it may be advisable to obtain an ultrasound. Remember that for purposes of dating, ultrasound results are less reliable after 20 weeks. Also, I have found that fundal measurements (per centimeter) are often very close to weeks, when taken between 16 weeks and 35 weeks. And I have discovered that adding exactly five months to the date when the mother feels the first good kick is an amazingly good predictor. (Do not use the reported "butterfly kiss" but an unmistakable kick.)

If you suspect a postterm baby, you may want to obtain a biophysical profile per ultrasound exam, which will offer information about the maturity of the placenta as well as amniotic fluid volume and bone maturity of the fetus. You may also want to obtain a serum estriol level, another diagnostic test for determining placental function, as well as have the mother tally fetal movements on a kick chart.

When it is established that true postmaturity is developing, every effort should be made to effect delivery. Careful monitoring of the fetus should be

(Continued on next page)

photo by Patti Ramos, digital art by Jennifer Rosenberg

paramount, especially during second stage, and the mother should be transported to a hospital for delivery should you detect any sign of fetal distress.

Tips & Tricks

Routine Urine Dip Sticks?

The routine search urine dip stick test at every prenatal has been challenged in the last decade. So many women show presence of albumin or glucose that the results are usually ignored unless there are other symptoms. Many are changing to a policy in keeping with the common international practice of testing urine only in the presence of symptoms of urinary tract infections, diabetes or pregnancy induced hypertension.

The more complex sticks include tests for ketones, leukocytes, blood, nitrates, etc. Many use the sticks as a screen for hidden (non-symptomatic) UTIs. But I think a better screen for asymptomatic UTI may be to send a sample for lab urinalysis rather than rely on dip testing for nitrates and leukocytes.

Because the research shows routine dip testing is inefficient, inaccurate and expensive, I follow the recommendations from the *Guide to Effective Care*, and I test urine only for indications or when there are symptoms. I no longer do the urine dip sticks at every prenatal.

Gail Hart, OR

Love the Baby Out!

Encourage lovemaking during pregnancy. The Japanese say, "Use the container so it's easy to open."

Aki Otani, Japan

Sweet Sounds

The same music a baby hears often while in utero may calm her during birth and beyond.

Tricks of the Trade Circle, Hawaii '96

Tipping the Pitcher

Think of a pregnant woman's bladder as a pitcher. When she pees, have her tilt forward, gently lifting her belly to the right and then to the left. Each time she'll get a little more out by "tipping the pitcher." This helps her relieve the discomfort of not being able to fully empty her bladder, which may also lead to urinary tract infection.

Lisa Goldstein, NC

Non-violent Induction

Our recipe for moms who are at term or past dates, and who are anxious for their babies to arrive, is a simple one: We tell them to go on a date with their husbands, have a glass of wine with dinner, then go home and make love. We remind them that semen is a remarkably effective prostaglandin enhancer and can be very effective in ripening the cervix. It is amazing how well this prescription works!

The second technique I use when it is becoming more important for the baby to be born is stripping the membranes. I am aware this method is losing favor, but I feel it is a lot safer than using Pitocin or prostaglandin gels. Labor usually ensues in about 72 hours and is enhanced by the couple's making love.

I still feel that the safest method of induction is castor oil. Many other induction methods, such as amniotomy, are irreversible and often lead to cesarean section due to "failure to progress" or time constraints for ruptured membranes. The worst things that will happen if the castor oil fails to bring on labor is that the mom will have some diarrhea and need some minerals replenished.

This castor oil recipe is not unpleasant for the mom and leads to good results: Blend 4 ounces of oil with just enough citrus juice (cuts the oil) to make it liquid. Have another glass of fresh juice, as well as a wash cloth drenched with hot water, at hand. Ask the mom to drink the castor oil mixture as quickly as possible. Then tell her to wipe out her mouth with the cloth to remove the oily residue. Next, have her rinse out her mouth with the fresh juice and spit it out. Finally, suggest she sit down to finish the rest of the juice slowly. The castor oil has no taste, it just feels awful, so this method really helps make it more palatable. The castor oil usually causes the bowels to empty within three hours. (We offer the mom "baby wipes" instead of toilet paper to prevent soreness.) Next, suggest the mom get into a very warm bath, and pour water over her abdomen. If a Jacuzzi is available, all the better! Contractions will usually begin while the mom is enjoying her bath.

Relaxation for Pregnancy and Labor

by Sabrina Cuddy, MPH

Relaxation sounds like something that should be easy, but for most of us, it takes a lot of practice to be able to relax enough to reduce pain in labor! It can take as much as three months to really train yourself or someone else to relax. The three important components to relaxation are the physical body, the mind and the emotional state.

The Physical Body

To relax your body, you need to be focused on the present (mind) and in a place where you feel safe (emotion). Start out learning to relax while you are somewhere you normally go to unwind—your favorite chair or your bed would be good choices. Later, you will want to practice relaxing in places that are less calm, such as while riding in the car or sitting in a noisy place. Practice letting go of your tension while in a variety of situations and positions: standing in line at the store, for example.

A good exercise to start with is called "tense and release." Get comfortable and travel through your body, tightening and then releasing each body part. Be sure to take enough time to really feel the relaxation as you let go. As an example, try your hands, one at a time. Make a tight fist and feel the different levels of tension as you let the fist go, very slowly allowing your hand to go totally limp. Try not to tense any body parts you are not working on at the moment.

(Continued on next page)

Next, try a technique called "progressive relaxation." This is just like tense and release, except you skip the tensing part. Focus on each part of your body and feel it totally relax before you go on to the next body part. You may find that you fall asleep at first, but try to stay awake until you have gone through your entire body.

Massage is very helpful and can be anything from gentle stroking with fingertips to the kneading motion we usually think of when we picture massage. It is a powerful tool for helping a woman when she is in labor.

The Mind

Imagery can help you focus on relaxation so that you do not start to think about the rest of your life and tense up again! While practicing progressive relaxation, try picturing yourself under a shower of warm water: the water washes the tension out of your body from your head to your feet.

In labor, mental imagery can be used to distract a woman from her contractions, or it can be used to help her tune in to what her body is doing. Different techniques will help different people, so be prepared for whatever happens by practicing both.

One of my favorite imagery exercises, called rainbow, can be used for practice, then condensed to a version that works very well for a 60-second contraction. Get physically relaxed, then have someone talk you through the exercise. The person guiding you will have you close your eyes and picture a movie screen. He or she will then ask you to visualize the colors of the rainbow, slowly showing on the screen one after another: red, orange, yellow, green, blue, indigo, violet, and finally fading to white, with the white light getting very bright.

Here is a sample color (you can use this as a script replacing the color name as you go through each color): "Picture before your eyes the color red. A bright red. Now picture an object that is red." Some women do better if the imagery is related to labor. You can have someone talk you through picturing your cervix open as the contraction increases in strength, bringing you closer to your baby! If you cannot picture your cervix, it may help to visualize it like a flower opening from bud to full bloom. Any imagery of things opening can help a mother open up and give birth.

Emotional State

For those assisting labor, if you can help the mother in labor stay calm, she will feel less pain. Emotional relaxation is greatly enhanced by providing an environment that feels safe to the mother. This often involves lowering the room lights, playing music that she finds familiar and relaxing, scenting the room with lavender (which has aromatherapy value for relaxation) or some other fragrance she likes, and keeping the temperature comfortable. Some women prefer natural daylight to darkness, so really listen to her preferences.

Some women in labor respond well to hearing poetry, Scripture and stories from their childhood, or stories made up about the new baby. For every woman, the presence of a supportive person in the room is a big bonus. If she gets to a point where she does not want you to touch her or talk to her, she will still appreciate that you are there and will respond to the calming sound of your regular breathing. It is very important for you to stay calm when you are with her!

For the mother, not only are relaxation techniques healthy to use in pregnancy, but they also can help you cope with the baby after it is born.

Among the many tapes available to help you learn how to relax and practice relaxing, I particularly like those from Source* recorded by Dr. Emmett Miller, a hypnotherapist. A good one to start with is "Letting Go of Stress," which features imagery exercises that take you on a trip to the beach. If you have been practicing relaxation already, you might want to go with more advanced tapes such as "Rainbow Butterfly" or "Source Meditation." If you have high blood pressure or another health issue, you might like to try "The Healing Journey."

How often should you practice relaxation? I recommend that you practice every night as you go to bed. In the third trimester, try to practice once every day by yourself and three to four evenings every week with your partner. I highly recommend doing a set of pelvic rocks at midday, lying down afterward to practice relaxing for about 10 minutes.

Stay relaxed and enjoy your pregnancy!

*Source catalogs and materials are available at 1-800-528-2737.

Tips & Tricks

Birth Plan Avoids Embarrassment

Any woman who is subjected to indignities at the hospital—questions about weight gain, sexually transmitted diseases, number of pregnancies, and so forth, asked in front of others—can report it to the director of nurses and the educational director at the hospital. One way to avoid this kind of problem in the first place is to have a birth plan that is written in sections.

The first segment can be for the prenatal practitioner with whom the woman will discuss aspects that are controversial. Another segment can be short and to the point for the admitting clerk; it can tell what the woman is comfortable answering in "public." A copy of this segment could also be given to the pre-admittance personnel so that it can be attached to her chart when she is admitted for her birth. The next segment, again short and to the point, is for the admitting nurse. Remember, they are busy, and some are opinionated or have an authority complex.

Roberta Gerke, CNM, MT

Packet Packaging

Package research-based information to present to parents and providers. Organize the packets by topic, such as VBAC, postdates, natural birth, cesarean and so forth. When there's a turn of events, information will be right at hand—no more scrambling!

Jill Cohen & Jan Tritten

Turn That Breech!

I read some while ago of a midwife who found it very effective to use a flashlight on the mother's abdomen in a very dark room to encourage a breech baby to turn. She would slowly move the light in the direction she wished to fetus to turn.

Rayner Garner (E-News)

Postdates vs. Postmaturity: An Overview

by Anne Frye, CPM

As I studied and researched the issue of postmaturity for volume I of my book *Holistic Midwifery*, it became apparent to me that much is claimed to be true about postmaturity that is flatly contradicted by recent research into placental function and pathology. This article will provide an overview of the postterm/postmaturity issue and attempt to clarify some of the questions that need to be kept in mind when assessing current postmaturity protocols and what you will do in cases of postmature pregnancies. Your understanding of this article will be greatly enhanced if you review my two-part article on maternal nutrition, which appeared in Issues No. 34 and 35 of *Midwifery Today*.

Postdates or postterm pregnancy is defined as a pregnancy that exceeds the 42nd week. In many obstetrical practices, being postdates is a high-risk category and increases the barrage of interventions that the medical model will force upon a woman until she gives birth. This is because a few babies from postdate pregnancies will exhibit postmaturity syndrome: a compromised baby possibly due to the extended length of pregnancy. This attitude assumes you have taken into account such variables as family history of length of gestation, parity and length of the menstrual cycle in arriving at an individualized due date, and now have a woman who is approaching 40 weeks or more.

Is the due date correct? In order to find out if a problem truly exists, the first thing to do is re-examine the due date. (For a full discussion of this, you might wish to refer to the chapter in *Holistic Midwifery* on "Calculating the Due Date," found in the Basic Skills section.)

Postdatism vs. Postmaturity Syndrome

In a well-nourished woman who salts to taste and drinks to thirst, pregnancy usually proceeds to term and often goes one to two weeks past the 40-week mark. In fact, 42 weeks may be the normal gestation for humans. When a well-expanded blood volume has stimulated a well-grown and well-nourished placenta, neither baby nor placenta will suffer before birth occurs. Fetal growth continues; fetal movement and heart rate variability maintain themselves normally; the volume of amniotic fluid is adequate; blood volume remains appropriately expanded providing optimal placental profusion; and everything is fine.

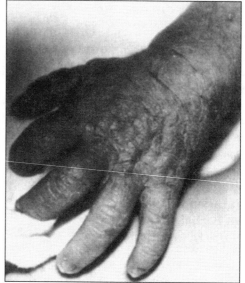
photo by Caroline E. Brown

Such a pregnancy may be postdates by the classic definition of the term, but it is not postmature. Most women assumed to be postdates have been misclassified based on an inaccurate due date. Their babies are quite healthy. In fact, congenital anomalies, infection and intrauterine growth retardation account for much of the perinatal mortality generally lumped into the postmature category. About 10 percent of babies are postdates, of which only 5 percent to 26 percent exhibit postmaturity syndrome. One study of 7,005 infants, which excluded babies from mothers with conditions known to affect fetal size, found the mean birth weight increased as pregnancy advanced. No babies weighing less than 2,500 grams were born after 42 weeks. No evidence of weight loss or lower weight for length was found. The study concluded there is a lack of convincing evidence that the postterm baby of a healthy mother is at increased risk of distress or nutritional deprivation.

While physicians talk about dysmaturity, at the same time they don't want pregnancy to go beyond 42 weeks for fear that the baby will grow too big! Obviously, a large healthy baby of a well-nourished mother is not suffering from intrauterine starvation. Furthermore, performing cesareans for "macrosomia" (defined as any baby larger than 4,000 grams or 8 pounds, 13 ounces) does not decrease the rate of asphyxia or injury.

When is there cause for concern? In any of the following cases, you may have to be more concerned about the possibility of inadequate blood flow to the placenta, the real culprit in creating a compromised baby, regardless of gestational age:

- Women who have been poorly nourished for reasons such as vomiting, nausea, poverty, and so on, for more than a week during the pregnancy; however, the placenta grows throughout pregnancy so any improvement in diet can be beneficial.

- Any woman who smokes or takes excessive amounts of poorly assimilated calcium supplements or antacids containing calcium during her pregnancy and has a marginal diet.

- Women who have had placental bleeding unrelated to previa, as this may

(Continued on next page)

indicate a poorly adhered placenta. Dietary improvement and vitamin E (up to 2,000 IU at the time of bleeding) can help strengthen the placental bed.

• Women experiencing no uterine activity (such as toning contractions) by the 34th week of pregnancy, or no cervical twinges or low menstrual-like sensations by 37 weeks. This can represent inadequate hormonal activity. Equinox Botanicals Prenatal Uterine Tonic, started at 34 weeks, can help to balance this out.

• Women who have had pituitary or hypothyroid disorders. Sometimes these problems are not evident until labor fails to begin. Watch for appropriate breast changes during pregnancy and adequate toning contractions without herbal assistance. (If there is a history of hypoactivity, glandular supplements may help; if hyperactivity has been a problem, homeopathic preparation of either pituitary or thyroid [3X potency] can be alternated every other day during the entire pregnancy to gently support the gland without overstimulation. Which supplement you use will depend upon the gland involved. Consultation with a naturopath is recommended.)

Anything which causes poor placental implantation, interferes with circulation to the placental surface, or otherwise leads to improper fetal nourishment can result in a situation that does not support a healthy pregnancy until birth and, therefore, what is termed postmaturity syndrome or dysmaturity in the newborn. In these cases you may get any of the following problems, depending upon the degree of severity: meconium staining; a baby with loose skin, appearing to have lost weight; little or no skull flexibility due to calcification of the bones; and a placenta inadequately supplied with blood to compensate for the lower oxygen supplied to the uterus during contractions.

These newborn problems were first described in a small study of 37 infants ranging between 285 to 325 days of gestation (41 weeks to 46.4 weeks). Clifford (1954) described three grades of severity, but the ages of the infants widely overlapped within each grade; no control infants were examined and no evidence that problems related to placental insufficiency was presented. In fact, postmaturity syndrome is not exclusively related to postdates babies, nor do its signs have clinical importance other than to demonstrate malnourishment of the fetus in utero. Those symptoms ascribed to postmaturity may simply be due to a baby with a degree of intrauterine growth retardation who has gone past term. The postdates babies at highest risk are those weighing less than 2,500 grams (5 pounds, 8 ounces), which is not surprising if poor maternal nutrition is the real problem. The most frequent cause of death in these cases is congenital malformation.

Placental Factors

A placenta compromised by inadequate blood flow from a poorly expanded blood volume or vasoconstriction of the uterine arteries (as might be the case in a smoker) results in a poorly nourished baby. While postmaturity has been commonly blamed on placental insufficiency, and felt to be the result of infarcts (dead spaces) and calcifications, these problems by themselves are not so serious if blood flow to the placenta is adequate. The fact that the villous surface of the placenta expands right up until birth

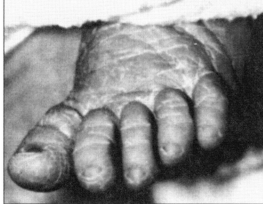
photo by Caroline E. Brown

(Continued on next page)

Tips & Tricks
Calculating Cycles & Due Dates

When women have unusual cycle lengths, I always calculate the due date from the estimated ovulation (conception) date, not the date of the last menses. Then I calculate the gestational age through the pregnancy from the estimated date of birth, not the last menstrual period. Still, there are ladies who make healthy babies "fast" and "slow," so the problem isn't entirely solved, but this certainly helps!
Cynthia Flynn, CNM, PhD (E-News)

When first speaking to a group of pregnant women, especially first-time mothers, I spend an extraordinary amount of time with them on calculating their due date. We know that statistically a first-time mother will need from 38 to 42 weeks and longer for her baby to be ready. I help them adjust their due date beyond the 40 week estimated due date, at least 10 to 14 days longer. Then I talk to them about the dangers of induction. I ask them if they think that any person or machine can tell them the exact day and hour their unique baby will be ready.

It is also important to talk about some of the foolishness some medical professionals are using to schedule birth, like "some women never go into labor on their own" (absolutely untrue); "your baby is overdue" (if you are a first-time mother that is what is supposed to happen); "your baby is too small" (a guess of a 5-pound birth weight in utero is most often shown to be incorrect when we actually have a baby to weigh); or one used often with older mothers, "your placenta is aging." I handle the last one by comparing the placenta to a refrigerator. Regardless of the age of the fridge, as long as we are filling it up with food it does not matter how old the fridge is. The placenta does not have an expiration date on it. Every time you eat you are nourishing the placenta and your baby.

Your body and your baby go through hundreds of minute changes in order to be prepared for birth. Forcing birth unnaturally can only lead to problems for both the baby and mother through the birth and after. Waiting for birth to start naturally will give them a faster, easier and safer childbirth.
Gail J. Dahl (E-News)

means that the placenta does not "get old" in the way it has been thought, and that any improvements the mother makes which increase blood flow to the placenta (improving her diet, quitting smoking, for example) will benefit the pregnancy until the end.

Many mainstream practitioners encourage women to take antacids (especially Tums) to relieve heartburn, feeling that they will get an "added benefit" because these products contain calcium. However, this calcium is not well assimilated, as is frequently apparent from looking at the placenta after birth. If an excessive amount has been taken, the placenta may be full of calcifications. Poorly assimilated supplements, hard (mineralized) drinking water or smoking can also cause excessive placental calcifications. The combination of many calcifications and a marginally expanded blood volume are a set-up for trouble. Furthermore, a calcified placenta is more fragile and more likely to break up during detachment after the birth. If a woman comes to you with such a history, you must take these factors into account. Bio-technical providers are also recommending aspirin for high blood pressure. Since aspirin and other salicylates interfere with prostaglandin production, this may increase the chances of a prolonged pregnancy as well.

Dealing With Postdatism in a Well-nourished Woman

First, recheck the due date and previous pregnancy history of the client and her mother (what was her mother's length of gestation?). Recurrent postdates pregnancies may be normal for a particular woman and are often seen among women in the same family. Check uterine size and fetal growth, contraction activity, cervical sensations, heart rate variability and reactivity, and amount of amniotic fluid at each prenatal. Have the mother keep a daily fetal movement chart (see *Understanding Diagnostic Tests in the Childbearing Year*, by Anne Frye). See her weekly until birth.

Make sure she continues to eat well and to drink plenty of clear fluids: six to eight glasses daily or more if she is thirstier or lives in an extremely dry climate. I suspect that some women unconsciously reduce their fluid intake at the end of pregnancy because the increasing pressure from the presenting part results in more frequent urination. In the normal situation, amniotic fluid volume is directly related to maternal fluid intake; it is therefore important that women know how vital it is to keep drinking. If all signs look good, relax and wait for labor to start. In my experience, some women who are fairly well nourished have reduced amniotic fluid volume when they carry to 43 weeks, with no other symptoms; attention to daily fluid intake should lessen this possibility. Less fluid or the suspicion of it calls for discussion of a Biophysical Profile test and diligent fetal heart monitoring in labor. Oligohydramnios correlates with fetal distress, probably due to cord compression. However, the amount of amniotic fluid does not correlate with outcome, and it is unclear to what extent reduced fluid is characteristic of prolonged pregnancy or when intervention solely for this factor is warranted.

Dealing With Postdatism in a Less-than-well-nourished Woman

In situations that may develop into true dysmaturity (postmaturity) syndrome—either from history, clinical signs, or intuition on your part or the mother's—monitor her at each prenatal as described in the previous section. Depending on your findings and the individual situation, you may also want to employ any of the following:

• Beginning at 36 weeks, have the mother record fetal activity daily and review this chart at every visit.

• At every prenatal assess the fetal heart rate for good variability and for accelerations with fetal movement. (See the chapters on "Fetal Activity Test" and "Assessment of Fetal Movement" in *Understanding Diagnostic Tests in the Childbearing Year*.)

• Give Equinox Botanicals Uterine Tonic for the four weeks before term, or at any time during the pregnancy if you suspect a problem. Other products can be used interchangeably with this tonic, as long as they do not contain pennyroyal.

• If, in spite of therapies, no uterine activity is present, have the mother do nipple stimulation starting at 38 weeks. This can be done by rolling the nipple end between the fingers or by applying gentle suction with a breast pump. If stimulation causes contractions longer than one minute in duration, stop that session at that point.

• To ripen the cervix, have the mother take three 300 mg doses of evening primrose, borage or black currant oil daily beginning at 36 weeks and continuing until birth.

• Starting at 36 weeks to 37 weeks, she should take three tablets daily of glandular pituitary extract, which may help to prime the pituitary gland to produce adequate oxytocin. (Do not use this if there is a history of hyperactive pituitary function. Instead use a homeopathic preparation of Pituitary [3X], one dose every other day throughout pregnancy.)

• Heterosexual intercourse provides prostaglandins in the form of semen. If the mother has a male partner and is so inclined, frequent sex will help ripen the cervix.

• At 36 weeks, begin the following homeopathic remedies: cimicifuga 12C, one pellet on Monday; caulophyllum 12C, one pellet on Wednesday; arnica 12C, one pellet on Friday. Continue to take each remedy once weekly as suggested until birth. This will help prime the uterus for the timely onset of effective labor and minimize physical trauma to mother and baby.

• If clinical evaluation suggests a problem or if the woman is past 42 weeks of pregnancy, do not hesitate to discuss a Biophysical Profile to assess fetal well-being. While prenatal testing is not by any means 100 percent reliable as to the condition of the baby, at least this test offers five variables from which to judge well-being, and also is fairly reliable if severe distress is discovered. If you feel it is advisable to attempt labor induction in a woman who has reached or passed term, refer to volume II of *Holistic Midwifery* or the postmaturity chapter in *Understanding Diagnostic Tests in the Childbearing Year* for suggestions.

Psychological Factors and Postdatism

For a variety of reasons, conscious or unconscious, a woman may be holding off her labor. She may be afraid she can't do it; she may be waiting for a friend or relative to arrive (or leave!). She may feel ambivalent about her birth choices or uncertain about her ability to mother or her relationship with her partner. In the midst of evaluating physical signs, be sure you are sensitive to emotional symptoms as well. In addition, there is the cultural stress of going beyond her due date. This fact cannot be dealt with in a vacuum and your relatively gentle interventions to encourage physiological readiness for labor will serve to insulate women, to a certain extent, from the medical hysteria in the larger society. A woman's feelings about these factors should be discussed as well. A solid relationship throughout pregnancy will provide the framework through which conflicts and problems can be expressed and released.

Helping the Mother Deal With Being Overdue

Inevitably, families and friends are anxious and excited when a woman nears her due date. When she carries beyond it, they can be real pests— to put it bluntly! Typically, people call on a daily basis, questioning the mother about any symptoms of labor and asking what the midwife has said or recommended. The best thing the mother can do is use an answering machine to screen calls or, if she can afford it, use the new device that lets her know the number of who is calling before she picks up the phone. In this way she can avoid some of this aggravation. With all the cultural hysteria over

(Continued on next page)

Tips & Tricks
Patience and Postdates

I was trained by Mary Ann Watson, CPM, QE, a direct-entry midwife with over 18 years' experience in homebirth. Her philosophy/protocols regarding induction questions are:

What if I never go into labor?
Women were designed to give birth. Gestation for each mother with each baby will occur at its own pace, just as labor progresses at its own pace. Just because the baby inside feels large enough to survive, it may need more time inside to develop a crucial system. No woman has ever been pregnant forever. Mary Ann continues weekly prenatal visits until the birth. As long as no complications arise, she does not risk out or induce women just because they are overdue.

What if my baby is too big?
Normal, healthy women do not grow babies they cannot birth. The species would have destroyed itself if this were true. Induction may also contribute to malpresentation. If the baby is allowed time to find a good birthing position, it will adapt to the pelvic inlet. Arbitrary induction may cause labor to begin before the baby is in a good position.

Should VBACs be induced?
Mary Ann's practice prior to coming to Kentucky was primarily VBAC births. She has an excellent record of successful VBAC births. Her VBAC moms are not induced and do not have a greater complication or transport rate than her other clients.

What if the placenta stops functioning?
Normal, healthy placentas do not just stop functioning 14 days past the due date. I myself have had one client go either three or five weeks overdue (she was unsure of her dates). Mary Ann has had clients confirmed at 30 days or more overdue. Those babies were fine, and those placentas were healthy.

Some women do try to induce themselves with herbal preparations, castor oil or some other home preparation. She firmly discourages this, for all the reasons above. Many of these induction attempts are not successful. One mother who was successful in inducing labor later regretted it. She had three productive, relatively short, labors. This fourth, induced labor was long, slowly productive and exhausting. She now discourages other women from trying to induce labor.

Our philosophy that birth is a natural process and our desire to allow it to progress with no intervention that is not absolutely necessary begins with good prenatal care and with accepting that labor will begin when it is time.

Candy Hall (E-News)

The best advice my midwife gave me in the last days of my pregnancies when I was beginning to feel impatient was, "The baby will come out when the baby is ready to come out." I think in most cases we need to stop hurrying the poor babies and give the mom some love and emotional support. My midwife also told me that during those last weeks and days, the baby's brain is developing. Realizing that it was an important time for the baby's development made it much easier for me to be patient.

K.L.M. (E-News)

If mom gets impatient and uncomfortable, it is our responsibility to counsel her to be patient and help her understand the reasons why patience is still the safest option. A safer option than worrying about "due dates" would be to ensure that mom has an optimum diet so that she and baby have optimum health when they go into labor.

Elaine (E-News)

Tips & Tricks
Due Dates

According to the medical literature, human gestation ranges from 36 to 44 weeks. That is a two-month range, not the due date plus or minus two weeks. The mean length of time plus or minus one standard deviation gives the 38 to 42 weeks range, with 40 weeks the average, or mean.

The mean has come to mean the right answer. Phooey! Here is an analogy: Few people actually have a 98.6 F temperature; that is an average. Some actually feel unwell if their temperature is 98.6 because their own body temperature is lower. Everyone has his or her own range. So it is with due dates.

I hate the whole idea of "due date." It is only a guess that creates expectation. The woman often circles that date on her calendar so she won't schedule any other appointments for that day. Better to teach women that the misery of late pregnancy is a natural motivation to want to go into labor, which is a natural progression from the joy of showing the sweet little belly that occurs in the early months. Teach them how to pay attention to their babies to know if things are OK in there. Babies will still play and respond inside even at the very end.

As a cranio-sacral therapy practitioner, I appreciate the power of intention and belief. When the health care provider gets worried about the length of gestation, that worry communicates to the woman, who may delay the start of labor longer because her adrenaline level can go up. Worry and beliefs are contagious. And we all know that adrenaline is the enemy of oxytocin!

So let's organize to keep pregnant ladies happy. Watch them with love, and for heaven's sake, let the baby come when it wants.

Nikki Lee (E-News)

postmaturity, the last thing a woman needs are family and friends adding to the stress.

Going overdue can be an anxiety-producing experience for a woman, especially if she is being seen by a medical model care provider. You can go a long way toward creating the space for labor to begin by being supportive and sensitive, and by having an intuitive "take" on her real risk.

References and further reading:

Boyd, M., et al. (1983). Fetal macrosomia: prediction, risks, proposed management. *Ob/Gyn* 61(16): 715-722.
Clifford, S. (1954). Postmaturity with placental dysfunction. *J. Pediatrics* 44(1): 1-13.
Fox, H. (1991, March). A contemporary view of the human placenta. *Midwifery* 7(1): 31-39.
Kilpatrick, Sarah, et al. (1993, January). Maternal hydration increases amniotic fluid index in women with normal amniotic fluid. *Ob/Gyn* 81(1): 49-52.
Nichols, C. (1985). Postdate pregnancy, Part I: A literature review. *J. Nurse-Midwifery* 30(4): 222-239.
Shearer, M., and Estes, M. (1985). A critical review of the recent literature on postterm pregnancy and a look at women's experiences. *Birth* 12(2): 95-111.
Sims, M., and Walther, E. (1989). Neonatal morbidity and mortality and long-term outcome of postdate infants. *Clin Ob/Gyn* 32(2): 285-293.

Emotional Factors in Prolonged Pregnancy
by Maryl Smith, CPM, LM

Begin early in pregnancy to accustom the mother to the idea that a term pregnancy lasts anywhere from 37 to 42 weeks. Only 40 percent of mothers will deliver within five days on either side of the due date, and about two-thirds deliver within 10 days. Important attention to the following will help a mother cope with prolonged pregnancy:

1. Reassure her that her body is healthy and working perfectly. Remind her that 60 percent of women have their baby after the due date.
2. Reassure her that her baby is healthy and wonderful.
3. Help resolve any difficulties sleeping.
4. Ask about her social contacts and family relationships.
5. Have her turn on the telephone answering machine.
6. Give her statements that can be repeated for self-reassurance.
7. Examine worrisome statements by friends and relatives.
8. Include family and friends in a prenatal.
9. Check for overexertion or the inertia of depression.
10. Has she cried? Express empathy.
11. Leave a stethoscope, Pinard horn or Doppler with a mother if she finds it reassuring to hear her baby's heartbeat. Instruct her on proper use, inviting a phone call when she wants your input and is using a Doppler.
12. Discuss preparation, fears and husband's feelings to clear charged issues.
13. Discuss pressure coming from family members with impending airline departure dates (one of my least favorite circumstances).
14. Discuss inducement of labor.
15. Have her plan moments of self-indulgence and relaxation.
16. Encourage her to talk to her baby.
17. Provide gentle labor encouragements such as homeopathics or five-week botanical formulas so that she feels she has some active control over her circumstances.
18. Draw her baby on her belly with a washable felt pen.
19. Rave about small cervix changes or any descent in station.

Labor

Important Things I've Learned About Birth and Midwifery

by Rahima Baldwin Dancy, CPM

WHILE I'VE ALWAYS known that "babies come out," the rest of these things I've learned in association with my longtime friend and midwifery partner of the last seven years, Valerie El Halta, one of the most experienced midwives in the country.

1. Babies come out!
2. Prenatal care is designed to help educate the woman and assess/prevent complications, but its main purpose is to develop a relationship of trust between the midwife and the mother, thus making the birth easier.
3. Certainty and absolute love on the part of the midwife make it unnecessary to work on most of the client's psychological problems.
4. There may be potential complications and emergencies. The midwife's job is to recognize such situations early and correct them (or transport if necessary) before they turn into real emergencies.
5. Sometimes the midwife's active intercession prevents a hospital transport—and whatever she does is always gentler than Pitocin drips, forceps or cesareans, not to mention the way babies are treated after the birth.
6. There is no such thing as "lack of progress" prior to 4 cm (accompanied by complete effacement with first-time mothers). Prior to 4 cm, mom is not yet in active labor, and it can take as long as it needs to, provided the midwife can keep her from becoming too tired.

If it is nighttime, it is usually better to rest the mother rather than try to stimulate contractions with walking, herbs and so forth. Respect the biological clock.

Several false starts can be associated with a posterior presentation, which should be addressed.

Dysfunctional uterine contractions

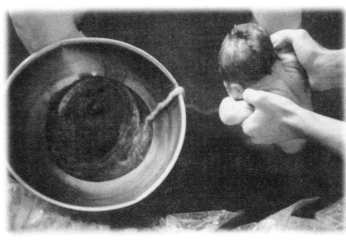
photo by Judith Halek

(contractions every few minutes that the mother finds painful but which are not dilating the cervix) can sometimes be knocked out with a warm bath, massage and a stiff drink; when they start again, the mother will be in good labor.

If a mother is very frightened, she may still only be 2 to 3 centimeters after several hours of strong labor. If the cervix is very thin and feels like a tight band, the midwife can "break it up" with her fingers, and the cervix will go to its true dilation (usually about 5 to 6 centimeters).

7. After 4 cm, there should be good progress, or the midwife should figure out the reason why not (lack of strong contractions, asynclitism, military presentation, posterior presentation, cord around the neck and so forth) and correct it.

Contractions can be stimulated by walking, nipple stimulation, a shower, emotional release and other "tricks of the trade."

If a posterior is suspected because of back pain and/or confirmed by feeling the fontanels, it should be corrected as early in labor as possible by putting the mother in the knee-chest position for 20 to 30 minutes, which helps bring the baby up out of the pelvis. The baby will usually rotate spontaneously. But if not, the midwife can push it up and turn it while the mother is in the knee-chest position. Once the baby is left occiput anterior (LOA) or right occiput anterior (ROA), the waters can be broken to assure its position.

If the baby's head is not flexed or is markedly crooked, the midwife can try pushing it up and turning it (using the knee-chest position if necessary). Climbing stairs or duck walking can correct problematic asynclitism.

Cord around the neck can be suspected if the head is not well applied to the cervix once the waters have broken, resulting in lack of progress (think of bungee jumping). Or you can suspect a wrapped cord if there are marked decelerations when the waters break. The cord can sometimes be heard down low with a Doppler. In such cases, if labor is allowed to progress slowly (sometimes keeping the mother lying on her side or wherever the heart tones are best), birth without fetal distress can be accomplished because the cord will stretch gradually (contrast this with the hospital's solution for lack of progress—Pitocin leading to fetal distress and a resulting cesarean).

8. When the mother is afraid, meconium may be evident. Without fear or a post-dates baby, you will very seldom see meconium in the waters (using the tub during labor also probably results in a lower incidence of the baby passing meconium).

9. About the only time you will see a
(Continued on next page)

healthy grand multip at risk is if she has overstretched uterine muscles (pendulous abdomen). This will keep the baby from engaging, resulting in danger of uterine prolapse, back pain and lack of progress because the baby isn't engaged or aimed at the exit. Use a prenatal cradle during pregnancy and have the mother labor lying down or with a belly wrap to help the baby stay vertical. Getting the head into the pelvis and breaking the waters can prevent cord prolapse (be sure to hold the baby in the pelvis from the outside while you break the bag to prevent it shooting up, thus increasing the risk of cord prolapse).

10. Expect a hand next to the face if you have uneven cervical dilation (the mother is complete except for cervix on the side) or if the mother has extreme pain right in front, just above the pubic bone. You may be able to try to move the arm from the outside.

11. If the mother is having trouble bringing the baby under the pubic bone despite strenuous pushing in a variety of positions (including squatting, which expands the pelvic diameters), the alley-oop position (McRobert's or "exaggerated lithotomy position") of bringing her knees back to her ears while she is flat on her back shortens the distance and brings the baby under the bone. An assistant on each side needs to bring the mother's legs back, even raising her sacrum off the bed if necessary, or clothespinning them (pushing in once they are back, to widen the pelvic outlet), depending on the nature of the problem. Alley-oop is especially useful if the mother has a narrow pubic arch because it utilizes the room in the back of the pelvis.

12. Shoulder dystocia can be expected if there is a really big baby with lack of progress in labor and slow birth of the head (when you have to birth the eyebrows, then the nose, then the mouth, then the chin). To prevent dystocia in such cases, birth the shoulders immediately on the oblique, before they have rotated and had a chance to lock behind the pubic bone. In 2,500 births with babies up to 13 pounds, 4 ounces, Valerie has never had a shoulder dystocia.

13. Babies do not need to be routinely suctioned at birth unless there is thick meconium or they don't start to breathe. Under normal circumstances, fluids are routinely expelled as they are born. This is facilitated by holding the baby face down, with the head lower than the body, as the baby is lifted onto the mother's stomach (hospital procedure always places the baby on its back, which keeps the baby from effectively spitting up). As long as the cord is still thick and blue, the baby is receiving as much oxygen as it did on the inside via the placenta and does not need to scream to take its first breaths.

14. Contractions, although often unfelt, continue after the birth; the placenta is almost always completely separated by the time of the third contraction (calculate how far apart contractions were in second stage). Putting the baby on or near the breast or using nipple stimulation provides positive backup. If first and second stages have gone normally, you need to trust that third stage will also go normally. After the requisite 10 to 15 minutes, put one finger on the uterus to tell when it is hard and ask the mother to give her placenta to you. The placenta is ready to be born then. This prevents problems such as concealed hemorrhage, letting the placenta get trapped by the cervix, etc. She will need to push, but tell her the placenta has no bones. You can use gentle cord traction or a squat if necessary. Because the cord has not yet been cut, sometimes the baby will signify when the placenta detaches by becoming fussy, as if complaining that it now has to be completely on its own.

Under normal circumstances the placenta does not "partially detach," and you may not see the "gush of blood" or "lengthening of the cord" described in the textbooks.

If a lobe is ingrown, or there is some other problem resulting in excess bleeding, or if the placenta isn't delivered as described above within 20 minutes, use Pitocin or herbs, put on a long sterile glove and feel what is going on (i.e., there will be some kind of anomaly: double-sized placenta that is trapped, extra lobe, strange surface, accreta, etc.).

When the placenta is delivered normally, it is not necessary to routinely massage the uterus; it will contract down by itself. If it does not and there is excess blood loss, use nipple stimulation, uterine massage, drugs or herbs for hemorrhage.

You can help lessen multips' painful afterbirth contractions right after birth by putting the side of your hand into the abdomen, just above the pubic bone, and lifting the uterus up.

15. By not cutting the cord until after the placenta is out, blood volume in the placenta and the baby remain more physiologically correct. The placenta delivers with fewer problems, and babies have less jaundice. We wrap the placenta in a Chux pad and tuck it in next to the mother, thus not interrupting the mother-baby interaction (doing this in the hospital prevents others from running off with the baby). By letting the mother request when to cut the cord, she lets us know when she is ready for the separation.

It is my hope that these suggestions will be helpful to other midwives.

Tips & Tricks

Secondhand

Being at birth can be messy, and supplies can be expensive. I ask my birthing couple to purchase as many used articles as possible, including large-sized men's shirts, sheets, towels, washcloths and so forth. I wash and dry them and store in a plastic bag as soon as they are dry. They're all ready for the birth!

Carrie Abbott, UT

Posterior Position

For a woman whose baby is posterior: If you have access to a swimming pool, float the woman belly down with the help of a flotation device—for hours, if possible. Follow with one hour of walking. Repeat this every day for several days. The baby should turn, and the mother can deliver easily.

Tricks of the Trade Circle, West Coast

Do Your Research

Order the booklet "Optimal Foetal Positioning" from Midwifery Today, Inc. Send $12.50, plus s/h. With the information in this booklet, combined with Valerie El Halta's techniques for turning a posterior baby, (*Midwifery Today* Issue 36) you won't have any more posterior babies.

Tricks of the Trade Circle, NY '96

Prolonged Labor: Past and Present

by Judy Edmunds, CPM, LDEM, LAM, RNC, CH

THE ELECTRICITY OF a hundred midwives charged the room. Sharing tips and techniques in a Midwifery Today tricks of the trade circle, the women kept returning to stalled labor—failure to progress. Many noted the frequent correlation to persistent posterior presentations with their protracted latent phase, requisite back pain and relative cephalopelvic disproportion (CPD). Some submitted ideas that were very hands-on and actually invasive, causing women subjected to them a fair bit of pain. Certain midwives listened with growing agitation despite assurances of success and stories of cesareans averted. "Women come to us to avoid intervention," they protested. "You're just substituting your own brand of meddling for medical management. Way too much interference! Why can't we just leave them be?" And finally: "What did women do 100 years ago?" The question hung in the air. Though we eventually moved on to other topics, the provocation remained.

What *was* done 100 years ago? What should our role be in trying to help? Where are we heading with our intrusions?

Of course, there is no simple answer. We each could name many situations and solutions, all correct in their own way. Many new birthing methods are indisputably detrimental, bizarrely technocentric and designed solely for caregiver convenience. But let's not throw the baby out with the bath water. We have the unique opportunity to marry the best of ancient ways with select modern innovations. When patience does fail us, wisdom and discernment may lead us to intervene judiciously, honoring the dignity of the process while offering strong but humble help.

In this context, let's examine the problem of prolonged labor. Historically, a woman was often given various potions to accelerate and strengthen contractions; her fundus wrapped down and manually compressed toward the opening, while prayers and chants implored divine aid. Evaluating heart tones or checking for cord entanglement was not customary. Concealed conditions such as elevated blood pressure, ketonuria, physical obstructions, abruptions or infection were often undetected. Primitive cesareans were extraordinarily risky and, fortunately, rare. Bloodletting might have been tried, as was forced vertex displacement for internal podalic version and breech extraction. Crude forceps were also used, symphysiotomies were performed and, as a last resort, fetuses were removed. Postpartum sepsis, which took the mother's life, was not uncommon.

Today these desperate tactics are no longer necessary. Modern obstetrics charges in with pharmaceutical reliance and surgical eventualities. While this approach may be overkill, it gets the job done. Lack of action may create its own problems. Sometimes, something simply must be done. In standing by indecisively, reluctant to interfere, matters may deteriorate to the point where heroics, however initially undesirable, become necessary. Thus, an optimum midwifery plan prepares for, expects and facilitates a simple birth while discreetly providing for any contingency necessitating intercession. The term "intercession" denotes benevolent assistance that is timely, effective and offered as a seamless aspect of one-to-one care, in a non-coercive, collaborative manner. One intervention does not usually precipitate another, but simply guides things back to a natural state of progression. The goal of any action should be to redirect labor back toward spontaneous and natural completion.

A successful birth plan requires careful preparation. Education during the prenatal period should inspire mutual respect and trust: the client takes in practical information while absorbing the midwife's firm confidence in birth. The midwife deepens and broadens her knowledge of the client, gaining insight

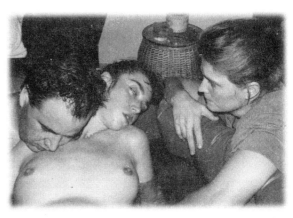

photo by Patti Ramos

into her personality and dreams for this birth, as well as notes her inner resources. Over the course of generous, unhurried prenatal visits, the woman comes to understand that the midwife genuinely cares for her and will not interpose frivolously. Situations that may require assistance are discussed beforehand, and informed consent is obtained in a setting where everyone is awake and clearheaded.

For instance, if I note a woman has a tendency toward posterior presentation, we discuss prenatally the implications for labor and steps we might take. By way of prophylaxis, I instruct the woman to spend time each day on her hands and (padded) knees, scrubbing floors, dusting low shelves or reading. I ask her to do pelvic rocks in this position, repeatedly arching her back high up into a stretch, then sinking her belly low to the floor. I model this and use a teddy bear to demonstrate how this requires a forward-facing baby trying to maintain its position, to brace upside down against a moving abdominal hammock, even as gravity tries to pull its top-heavy back around. The arching serves to further dislodge the baby's back from conforming to the mother's inner spine. Usually, the baby rather quickly finds an occipitoanterior (OA) position easier to sustain.

(Continued on next page)

Tips & Tricks

Gardening Basket

A gardening basket is useful for carrying essentials to a birth. The center of the basket can be used for storing gloves and gauze. The little elasticized side pockets around the outside of the basket can carry the bulb syringe, Delee, a squeeze bottle each of olive oil and betadine scrub, cord clamps, blood tubes, syringes and needles, and homeopathics. The basket can go right into a larger all-around equipment bag. During the birth it can go wherever the midwife goes, and her essentials are always at hand.

Marguerite Epstein, Internet

Easy Setup

Set up all your birth supplies in the placenta bowl. That way, if the mother changes her mind about where she intends to deliver, the equipment can easily follow her. I usually have two setups: the very important supplies, and the less important things. They can be combined into one bowl for third stage, and the second bowl is used for the placenta.

Unknown, America Online

Put a Tablecloth in Your Birthkit

A good-sized plastic tablecloth with a flannel back is a handy addition to your birthkit. You can toss one down just about anywhere—over a couch, chair, bed, or carpet. I put the plastic side down; because it is slightly textured it won't slip around as Chux or other plastic sheeting will. The flannel side is more comfortable than a Chux under the mother, won't rip, has no seams that will leak, and covers a large area. Because of their size and weight, mothers can move around without the tablecloth bunching and tearing like a Chux. They wash well, and can be reused. To top it off, they cost only a few dollars.

Gail Hart, America Online

Arnica for Tissue Elasticity

Arnica oil helps a woman's perineum stretch. When a woman's labia and perineum swell, give her oral arnica. You can see the tissue deflate in front of your eyes.

Tricks of the Trade Circle, NY '96

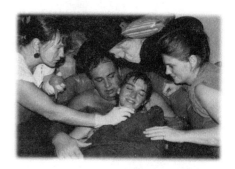

photo by Patti Ramos

Should labor commence with baby occipitoposterior (OP), time spent early on in deep knee-chest position, with widespread legs, may effect rotation. Other tricks to consider are duck walking, stair climbing with one leg abducted, lunging, quartersquatting or hula-style belly dancing. If these don't work, consider the uncomfortable intervention of internal manual conversion to anterior. Invasive? Very. And effective. Sure, many women push out wee ones sunny-side up with little fuss. I am convinced that multips who have ample pelvises with a history of happy births can do positively anything! However, the diminutive mom with a large baby, previously sectioned for failure to progress with a smaller, persistent posterior babe, is a poor candidate for watchful waiting. By getting close to our clients, we learn who would benefit from assertive action and whom we can simply sit on our hands with. Though not often needed, this is an example of a strongly interventive, briefly painful technique that may avert an even worse outcome: a brutal, protracted, traumatic labor with a surgical conclusion. Isn't that a worthy goal?

Labor marathons are often rooted in emotional discord. Fostering loving trust and loyal, determined commitment will usually see you through. As long as nutrition and hydration are offered freely, and vital signs remain reassuring, labor may take as long as it needs to. I don't believe there is a time limit. Families know we will turn toward surgical options only in cases of absolute need.

Unfortunately, caregiver fatigue, physician distress or boredom also lead to surgical interventions. The midwife transports because she is exhausted or inadequately prepared; the doctor proposes surgery out of his own burden of fear and expected role as deliverer. Tired and fed up with the whole mess, the family goes along with anything just to get it over with. Interventions at these times are not medically necessary, but under the duress of the situation, it seems like the best choice. This sort of decision is one that many later regret.

Our jobs are to blend diligent overseeing with sincere encouragement, massage, herbs or homeopathy, hydrotherapy, supported ambulation, music, prayer and rest. Studies validate these complementary modalities. When we have tried everything, we may still bring in fresh attendants or call for advice. We don't throw in the towel until we've tried absolutely everything and maybe even try something new. Only then will we know that we gave it our very best, so if something is really wrong, we will be grateful for that medical miracle.

A skillful midwife is more than a friendly handmaiden with monitoring tools and an ability to call 911. While I find infatuation with automated birthing repugnant, neither do I want to be the limited midwife of the past. Solidly grounded in contemporary knowledge and appropriate technology, I thrill at using new research to outwit complications, sharing methods with sister midwives around the world, finessing botanical combinations to surpass antibiotics' effectiveness, and refining manual approaches to problems to which others apply scalpels. I'm glad my Doppler amplifies fetal heartbeats for all to hear through even the thickest of abdomens, while mom rocks herself to her favorite music on hands and knees, her husband murmuring endearments in her ear. Once in a great, long while, I'm even glad for synthetic concoctions such as Pitocin. Having these modern tools available allows me to practice old-fashioned, high-touch, low-tech caring seasoned with the fruits of science.

May each of us draw intelligently from our myriad options, weaving together our own unique, specialized blend of knowledge for the fullest reproductive success.

Preventing Prolonged Labor

by Valerie El Halta

FAILURE TO PROGRESS—the most common reason for a cesarean—often really means a care provider is admitting frustration and impatience with a woman's labor. This is especially true if the woman is not laboring according to Friedman's Curve. Of course labor should progress reasonably. But there are more landmarks of progress than cervical dilation only. For instance, when a baby has a $15^{1/2}$ inch head, a mother will certainly need more time for molding to occur, and forcing a more rapid delivery will only cause harm to mom and baby.

Cephalohematoma, excessive caput formation and bruising might well be expected from forcing this larger baby through the pelvis, and some decelerations of heart tones would probably occur as well, from head compression. The mom will suffer from tearing and bruising of tissues that would have sufficiently stretched, given enough time. Progress may be marked by further descent, more effacement and softening of the cervix, or by noticing that the mother has become more able to deal with her environment and her contractions, allowing further progress to take place. There may be psychological reasons for slowed progress as well as physiological.

Let's examine the most frequent situations that lead to transport of the laboring woman to the hospital and learn to assist with these situations before they become complications. The following are the most common factors that occur before the diagnosis of failure to progress is made.

Possible Cephalopelvic Disproportion (CPD)

How often is this diagnosed as a reason for lack of progress when the baby's cephalo is nowhere near the pelvic to disproport? Although this is a possible condition, I believe it is relatively rare. I have probably seen only three true cases of CPD in my career. One stands out in my mind, since there was no arrest of labor until the beginning of second stage. When I probed more deeply to find the cause, I found a real deformity of the sacrum, which prevented the baby's descent past the inlet, which was adequate. Most other diagnoses of CPD are probably associated with arrest of labor due to a posterior or asynclitic presentation. Remember: Unless past term to the point that the plates are fixed and immobile, a baby with a large head can usually squeeze through just fine if time is allowed for adequate molding.

Malpresentation

I am not including here either the breech, which I consider a variation of normal, nor a complete transverse lie, which occurs before labor begins and should have been diagnosed long before there is failure to progress. I would like to address, however, presentations that may affect progress such as asynclitism, incomplete flexion, military, brow and face presentation, and of course, posterior.

The assumption is often made that when any of these situations occur, it is because the woman has an inadequate or smaller pelvis. Quite the contrary. Malpresentations of the fetal head most often are due to the woman's having an adequate to ample pelvis and a smaller baby who can move around freely. The most difficult to facilitate are those sweet little 6-pound babies with compound arms who are sucking their thumbs and kinking their heads out of alignment to the pelvis. The 9 and 10 pounders have just enough room to emerge correctly, having no room to play.

Asynclitism

Asynclitism is diagnosed when the suture lines of the fetal skull are not felt to be aligned exactly halfway between the symphysis pubis and the sacrum. If the baby's head is tilted up toward the pubic bone, it is called anterior asynclitism; if tilted toward the mother's sacrum, it is a posterior asynclitism. If the baby is not deeply engaged in the pelvis, the head may be adjusted by the midwife's manually lifting the baby's head upward if posterior or moving it downward if anterior. Having the mother climb up and down a flight of stairs when available may easily correct the asynclitism. If no stairs are available, suggest that she duck walk: while being supported, the mother bends her knees, broadens her stance, and walks, swaying from side to side, rotating her hips out and forward. Another trick, as demonstrated by Penny Simkin, is to have the mother place one foot on an elevated surface, with the lifted foot higher than the other knee. This position is held for several contractions and then the alternate leg is elevated.

I once had an interning midwife who thought the stair thing was really silly. When she returned to her practice, the second woman she was assisting had a marked lack of progress, and when it was determined that the baby was asynclitic, the midwife thought, "Well, let's try it," since the mom was on the second floor of her home. "Stuck" at 6 centimeters, the mom made it down the stairs and promptly delivered her baby right on the stairs, halfway back up! These techniques will assist in repositioning the head in cases of incomplete flexion and military presentation as well. Don't be afraid to use your hands to adjust those crooked little heads.

Posterior Labor

Many of the women who come to us desiring vaginal birth after cesarean have suffered a previous cesarean for failure to progress and CPD, and yet, when we receive the woman's records, the postoperative diagnosis usually confirms the posterior lie. It is my experience that with appropriate diagnosis and minimal intervention this condition can be corrected by assisting the baby to rotate as soon as it is diagnosed. Many times the position is not diagnosed until labor is advanced and progress arrested.

The incidence of a posterior presentation occurring at the onset of labor is 15 to 30 percent, and many such babies rotate spontaneously to an anterior position.

(Continued on next page)

When the pelvis is adequate, a posterior baby may be born face up with little or no difficulty. However, because we are unable to guess at the onset of labor what the possible outcome will be, I feel it imperative that every effort be made to avoid both a long and difficult labor and possible necessary operative intervention by early diagnosis and correction of the position.

At the onset of labor, it is important for the midwife to assess the position. It is relatively simple to assist the rotation of the baby when the mother is in early labor and very difficult once labor becomes advanced.

Assisting Anterior Rotation During Labor

When it is verified that the baby is in a posterior position, the first thing I do is have the mother assume and maintain a knee-chest position for approximately 45 minutes. Although this position is not the most comfortable one for the mother, it is very effective because it allows the baby more room in which to rotate. I find that the mother tolerates this position very well if she is not in advanced labor. We make sure she is well supported by plenty of pillows and give her lots of encouragement and emotional support. Often, while in the knee-chest position, the contractions become more regular and more effective, which also assists the baby's rotation.

If the mother cannot tolerate the knee-chest position for as long as necessary to turn the baby, we alternate by placing her in an exaggerated Simm's position—lying on the left side, two pillows under the right knee, which is jackknifed, left leg straight out and toward the back.

Every effort should be made to avoid rupturing the membranes, because the pillow offered by the forewaters gives a cushion on which the baby's head may spin more easily. Furthermore, if the waters break before the baby has rotated to the anterior, it is possible that sudden descent of the fetal skull will result in a deep transverse arrest!

If labor is more advanced when the posterior is identified, say 4 to 5 centimeters, it may be helpful while the mother is in the knee-chest position for the attendant to place her hand in the mother's vagina and gently lift the head, somewhat disengaging the head and allowing it to turn to anterior.

If the posterior has not been discovered until complete dilation, or if the above methods have not been applied in early labor, the baby's head may still be turned to make delivery more likely. Again, placing the mother in a knee-chest position, with knees slightly apart, the midwife may place her hand into the woman's vagina. Remember your hand is smaller than the baby's head. Attempt to lift the head up by grasping the head firmly, waiting for a contraction and turning the baby into an anterior position. As soon as the head is correctly positioned, hold on tight and when the uterus contracts again, urge the mother to push very hard! If the amniotic sac has not previously ruptured, rupture it now. This will assure that the position remains fixed and the baby will usually be born very rapidly. This procedure is both safe and sane, yet it must be acknowledged that it will take some physical strength to turn this recalcitrant little head against the force of a good contraction.

Brow Presentation

A Lebanese woman came to us when she was about 36 weeks into her second pregnancy. We were able to give her one prenatal visit before she went into labor at 37 weeks. Her first baby had been born in France and had weighed more than 8 pounds. Having had a difficult birth and determined not to repeat the experience, she severely restricted her diet, hoping to have a smaller baby. Of course, this only assured a premature baby! She labored well until she approached second stage. We had not done many vaginal exams because they distressed her, and since she was progressing normally, we just stayed with her, took heart tones and waited. We were sure the baby would be born quickly, and as she began to have good bearing down contractions, we prepared to receive her baby. We checked her and found her complete, but didn't really investigate the baby's head position. After an hour of second stage, there was no sign of the baby at the door. I told her it was important for me to check her again and that I needed to stay long enough to assess the suture lines and determine what was delaying her baby. I suspected a nuchal cord or hand. I found the baby was presenting with his brow.

This was my first brow presentation in about 2,000 births, so when I recovered from the surprise, I went immediately to my bible on presentation and position—*Human Labor and Birth,* by Oxorn and Foote—and turned to "brow presentation." I read the chapter and felt my diagnosis was correct. We returned to the birth room and encouraged her to keep pushing. Hands and knees, squatting, one foot elevated, duck walking—we tried it all. After three hours of extreme effort on the mother's part, the baby appeared on the perineum and was born over an intact perineum. He had very good APGAR scores but the poor little thing looked like an alien. He weighed only 6 pounds and had a normal-sized head, which was very molded. As we left the mom and baby to nestle, we were very relieved he had been born and was doing so well. I went back into the library to read again the chapter on brow presentation and noticed there was another page that I had not read.

"Prognosis: Brow Presentation" (Oxorn and Foote)
Mother: Passage of a brow through the pelvis is slower, harder, and more traumatic to the mother than any other presentation. Perineal laceration is inevitable and may extend high into the vaginal fornices or into the rectum because of the large diameter offered to the outlet.
Fetus: Fetal mortality is high. The excessive molding may cause irreparable damage to the brain.

Their recommendation in most instances of brow presentation is to do a cesarean as soon as it is diagnosed. Sigh!

I cannot emphasize strongly enough how important it is to make early assessment of the mother in labor. As in a posterior presentation, the brow may also be adjusted with little effort if found in early, or at the beginning of, active labor. At this point, the adjustment is made manually and is not painful for the mother, whose contractions are such that she can still relax. This is intercession! If manipulations are necessary at a later stage of labor, they

(Continued on next page)

will be painful, the mother has greater difficulty cooperating and relaxing, and operative intervention may become necessary.

Face Presentation

While brow presentations are extremely rare, occurring 1:3,000 to 1:1,000, or under 1 percent, face presentations may occur 1:250. While traumatic, the face presentation may be delivered safely as long as the position is anterior. The posterior face presentation—baby's body toward mother's back—is very difficult, if not impossible, since the baby's head is forced back upon its shoulders, and the head cannot come into the pelvic outlet. (It is as if the head and shoulders are descending as a unit.) Again, early diagnosis is imperative to assure the best outcome. I have encountered four face presentations in my 20 years of practice. I was able to correct the position in three instances and successfully assist with the delivery of the fourth.

Basically, two methods can be used in correcting the face presentation. First, the baby may be repositioned by external manipulation. In a manner similar to that of performing external version for a breech presentation, the baby must be disengaged and turned. This requires two sets of hands. The mother should be placed in a supine position with her hips elevated. One caregiver attempts to disengage the baby's head by lifting it upward (if not possible externally, then vaginally), while placing the other hand against the breech, causing the baby's body to flex. Another person places her hand against the baby's chest via the maternal abdomen and presses inward, further assisting with flexion. The literature addressed to obstetricians states that this can be done only at complete dilation with ruptured membranes. I highly disagree, since intact membranes and sufficient amniotic fluid will greatly increase the likelihood of success because the baby is able to move more freely. Attempting any version with broken waters greatly increases the risk of causing placental abruption, cord compression or prolapse, and fetal distress. Two of the three face presentations that I was able to reposition were done in this manner. The third was assisted by the second method, which is to place the mother in a knee-chest position, wait for up to 45 minutes to allow the baby to reposition spontaneously, and then manually lift the baby out of engagement and reposition the head vaginally. Caution: If you are able to successfully correct the face presentation with the first method (abdominal version), the baby will now most likely be posterior. If you utilize the second technique, the baby will not only become a normal vertex presentation, but will be able to rotate more easily into an anterior position.

Uterine Atony

If a malpresentation is not discovered, or other factors contribute to a long, nonprogressing labor, the uterus resumes with a good outcome if the mother is allowed to rest and labor is not forced to proceed. There have been cases of stalled labors that have been oxytocin augmented without remedying the cause, and they have resulted in uterine rupture. If there is no malpresentation or any other contributing factor (or they have been resolved), and the fetus is in no distress, the mother should be allowed to rest as long as necessary. She should be encouraged to eat and drink high carbohydrate, nourishing foods. If she is dehydrated and an IV is not available (or permissible), try giving potassium and electrolyte fluids both orally and by rectum, per enema bag. To stimulate contractions before mother is well rested will only lead to further complications, such as the development of constriction rings, fetal distress and third-stage difficulties.

Incoordinate Uterine Action

Incoordinate uterine action is a phenomenon that may occur in primipara labor. It is rare and difficult to diagnose and is often mistaken for failure to progress or assumed to be false labor. It is important that this condition be diagnosed, since the mother may soon become frustrated and disillusioned by her lack of progress. This can lead to numerous complications, such as maternal exhaustion, dehydration, constriction rings and so forth. Incoordinate uterine action presents as

(Continued on next page)

Tips & Tricks

History of Precipitous Labor

Make sure your midwife is called at the first signs of labor or impending labor (backache, bloody show, etc.). Even two hours is plenty of time if the midwife is not a hundred miles away.

Also, have a delivery kit ready at home and have your midwife review how to assist in the birth, support the perineum and stimulate the baby if necessary. Your partner will feel more comfortable if these basics are reviewed in the event the midwife does not arrive in time.

Anon. (E-News)

Just rely on planning. If your water breaks, call everyone immediately. You can even plan to have a family member stay with you for a few days before your due date. I learned that unnecessary worry does nothing.

Deana Sodders (E-News)

Have a (doula) friend who is familiar with emergency childbirth with you.

Chava Weiman (E-News)

Nurse's Watch

A nurse's watch enables you to glance at your watch no matter what your arms are doing. The watch is attached to a brooch-pin by a little chain. They withstand water, etc., very well and don't get near the site of the birth, meaning they neither collect material nor get a chance to contaminate. They are generally available at any jeweler's upon request.

Unknown, AOL

Comforting Sounds

During long labor sitting when either you, the mother, or both of you are dozing, wear something that jingles so that the woman knows as she drifts in and out of sleep that you are close by.

*Tricks of the Trade Circle,
1996 Pacific Rim Conference*

Aromatherapy

Misting a few drops of Rose Absolute mixed in water relieves tension in the birthing scene.

Judy Edmunds, WA

painful, frequent though irregular contractions that do not cause either effacement or dilation. Artificial stimulation of uterine contractions such as amniotomy or oxytocics do nothing to improve the contractility of the uterus, and the result is often cesarean section. When a woman has had this condition previously, she will often report that she never got past 2 centimeters, despite a lengthy induction.

When this condition is suspected, it is very important for malpresentation or posterior presentation to be ruled out because symptoms may be similar. The diagnosis may be confirmed by the attendant touching the cervix during a contraction and noting that there is no tension of the cervix during the contraction. The uterus contracts in the fundus but not in the lower uterine segment, or one side of the uterus may contract and not the other. Another variation is inverse—the contraction begins in the lower uterine segment rather than in the fundus. All these conditions are termed incoordinate. When this condition is suspected or conclusively diagnosed, the only effective treatment is to stop the contractions, and rest the mother for a period of time. When contractions resume spontaneously, the condition will be resolved and labor will progress normally. In the hospital, the mother may be given Valium or other drugs to stop the contractions, allowing her some rest. I have been successful in resting the mother by giving her two grams of calcium and allowing her to take a small amount of alcohol followed by a warm bath. Once the contractions are stopped and the mother is able to get some sleep, labor usually resumes in a normal pattern.

Maternal Exhaustion

When the attendant is vigilant in assessing the progress of labor—making sure there are no impediments to normal progress—and the mother is encouraged to be active, is well fed and is well hydrated, this condition should never occur. It is important that the mother be encouraged to rest and sleep as much as possible in very early labor. I often joke with a first-time mother who is preoccupied with watching the clock that no woman has ever missed her birth by sleeping through it. If exhaustion has occurred, labor will slow down, and inertia and constriction rings may lead to operative intervention. The risk of maternal hemorrhage increases, as well as the possibility of subinvolution with excessive bleeding and postpartum infection.

Maternal Hypoglycemia

Due to the increased stress of labor, the mother's stores of blood sugar diminish rapidly. Hypoglycemia is probably the most frequent cause for slow progress in labor, as well as increasing maternal irritability and difficulty in dealing with contractions. It is important for the mother to be fed during labor. I prefer to offer her high protein milk shakes to keep her blood sugar levels up. Giving fruit juices during labor is not recommended, since they may cause hyperacidity leading to heartburn and vomiting, which will heighten the problem. When the woman is not on an IV, it is important that she be given high glucose drinks immediately following birth, usually fruit juices of her choice.

Cervical Dystocia

There are several causes for primary cervical dystocia. Simple failure of the cervix to efface and dilate (achalasia of the cervix) and abnormal rigidity of the cervix and cervical conglutination (the lips of the os are adhered) are the pathological reasons. Dystocia may also be caused by scarring from a previous birth, from artificial cervical opening, or from injury to the cervix from operative intervention when a positive Pap smear has suggested cancer. A recent study regarding birth control pills has shown that a nullipara who has been on the pill for some time may have a rigid cervix as well. This does not seem to affect the multipara who uses the pill.

Cervical Adhesions

It is not unusual to find hard spots on the cervix during examination of a woman in labor. If the woman does not have condylomas, most often what you are feeling are small cervical scars from previous births or gynecological procedures. The use of instruments for dilating the cervix or delivering the baby often cause small tears to occur, as well as do women pushing their babies out prematurely (before complete dilation). These adhesions most often will break down during the active phase of labor. If you feel they are causing a lack of progress (the woman remains at 5 to 6 centimeters for more than an hour), you might consider simply pressing the adhesion against the presenting part during a contraction. You will feel the adhesion break up under your finger. This causes no pain and readily resolves the problem. There may be a spot of blood as this is done, but this is of no concern. The labor will usually progress rapidly after the adhesion is gone.

Psychological Factors

This topic alone could easily fill several chapters! Years ago, when I was first studying midwifery, I first heard the comment that "birth is basically a head trip." I believe this is true. If there are significant psychological problems, which may negatively impact labor and birth, it is important that these are discovered and acted upon before the time of birth. If the mother needs counseling or psychiatric help, the time to get it is before labor begins. From the simplest notion ("I can't have my baby until after my sister's bridal shower") to complicated issues regarding abuse or anger, all are paid attention to by the observant, caring midwife. Unresolved issues will come up during labor, possibly preventing labor from happening.

Tight Nuchal or Short Cord

When women think of complications, the most common question that arises is, "What if the cord is around the baby's neck?"

A nuchal cord is present in about a third of all deliveries and usually presents no problem. The issue, therefore, is not if the cord is present, but whether it is able to function in its delivery of blood and oxygen to the fetus during labor and delivery.

When there is a deceleration of the fetal heart beat at about 6 or 7 centimeters, I immediately suspect a tight or short nuchal cord. At this point in labor, the baby is beginning its descent and any constriction of the cord will become apparent. This is the most important time for listening to heart tones. If declarations are heard, we first change the mother's position to either hands and knees or to a left side lie. Nothing should be done to accelerate labor at this point! The cord will stretch if given enough time. Often, this change in maternal position is enough to correct the problem—the fetal heart rate returns to normal and we continue with the labor. If repositioning of the mother does not immediately allow the heart tones to resume to normal, I may go in and gently lift the baby's head, reducing the strain on the cord. If these measures do not allow the fetal heartbeat to resume to normal, do not continue with the labor. Transport the mother!

If the cord is not nuchal or shortened, it may be compressed, as in a hidden prolapse, by a leg, shoulder or other part. Since we cannot be sure of the problem, a good rule of thumb in dealing with bradycardia is to know that three separate episodes of decelerations of the fetal heartbeat are definitive of persistent, recurring bradycardia and, if this is the case, the woman should be transported to the hospital. She should be transported in the position that most positively affects the heart tones. If the cord is indeed very short or otherwise compressed, it may be necessary to transport as with a cord prolapse—with the mother in a knee-chest position and the caregiver's hand elevating the baby's head during transport.

If, as is usually the case, the fetus responds well and there is no further bradycardia, it may be expected that the birth will proceed normally. However, be prepared for infant resuscitation. Even if you have only had one episode of fetal bradycardia, there probably have been others that you have missed. Be sure to monitor heart tones again very often, if not continuously during the crowning and actual delivery of the baby, in case the birth needs to be hastened. When the baby's head is born, check for the cord around the neck and immediately assess if there are multiple loops. If the baby does not spontaneously emerge, it may be necessary to clamp and cut the cord, freeing the baby and allowing the body to be born. If as is usual the cord is singly looped, I advise that it be lifted over the baby's anterior shoulder rather than pulled over the head, as a short or overstretched cord is likely to separate from the placenta.

On rare occasions, the cord may separate from the placenta before the baby is born, or immediately after. A hemostat must be placed at the infant's umbilicus immediately because even a small loss of blood will be detrimental to the baby. Clamping the maternal side is of secondary concern because the blood coming from the cord is fetal. Wait for the normal period of placental separation and deliver by Brandt Andrews maneuver. If the separation has occurred at the placenta (it will most often be due to velamentous or Battledore insertion), and there is no cord for traction, the placenta may be delivered through maternal effort, with the attendant pressing down on the uterus toward the mother's spine to facilitate delivery. Never apply downward, fundal pressure because this will cause the uterus to prolapse or invert.

When there has been a short or nuchal cord, it is not unusual that a gush of blood accompanies the birth, since the placenta may have become partially separated from the uterine wall.

Expect some discoloration of the baby's face, since the tissues have been suffused. Explain to the parents that this is normal and doesn't indicate a heart defect. The baby has simply suffered from lack of oxygen.

Compound or Nuchal Arm

This occurs so frequently that it is considered fairly normal. Yet, when all other causes for hangups of labor have been eliminated, compound or nuchal arm is likely the cause. When suspected, the baby's elbow or hand may often be palpated just above the symphysis. The attendant may actually be able to cause the baby's hand or arm to retract by gently and firmly putting pressure against it externally and moving it away.

This is much easier to accomplish if the mother is submerged in water. Upon vaginal examination, I have found the hand at the side of the head or even over the head, and have been able to cause it to withdraw by simply poking at the fingers. The problem may not be discovered
(Continued on next page)

Tips & Tricks

Early Doula Attention

I began telling clients to call me very early in labor rather than wait for active labor as many had been doing. Why? When they deal with early labor on their own they often spend a lot of time worrying and getting scared and thus feel more pain than necessary early on. Not only is that early part of labor less productive, but it's also longer when a woman spends that time getting more and more tense.

So I tell them to call me when it first starts to get uncomfortable, even if the contractions are only 20 minutes apart. I go, help them settle down and quit focusing on the contractions. I often send them to bed (at night) or have them eat a snack if they've stopped eating. I might show them a few techniques dad can use to help mom with the contractions as they curl up together in bed or snuggle up on the couch. Then I leave them alone if it seems appropriate and tell them I'm going to take a nap in another room. This way they still have their privacy but also have the security of knowing someone is close. It really removes the fear—and since I work with women who birth in the hospital there's usually a lot of fear in the first part of labor.

Jennifer Rosenberg, Doula (E-News)

Humor and Labor

When the mother is closed down to you, instead of making suggestions, ask her what she wants. I also say obviously male things to make the woman laugh. That releases any tension she is holding.

Jerry Carrick, EMT, CA

Even a forced smile releases endorphins, the body's natural pain medicine that is similar to morphine. When we are with a birthing woman who is in pain, it may help to tell some good jokes—or even some not so good ones, especially in early labor. Carry a joke book in your birth bag!

Marianne Manley, RN, CNM, CA

Tips & Tricks

Hidden Tools

When I toured a birthing unit in Poland (see *Midwifery Today*, Issue 43), I noticed that the midwives kept the "scary" tools they might need in an emergency in a plain, unremarkable rolling drawer set away from the area rather than out in plain view. This small consideration kept the mothers from being frightened and intimidated.

Jan Tritten, OR

A Cool Solution

In late labor, women are often miserably hot and sweaty, even in air-conditioned environments. Hospitals usually don't allow the use of electric fans, and rural homebirth clients may not even have electricity. I always carry a folding metal and paper fan, the kind that costs a dollar or less. This small, simple tool can provide real comfort to a hardworking woman—plus it can give a nervous family member a useful job.

Catherine Feral

Chill Out

If the birthing mom is hot (from heating pad, hot packs, water, fever and so forth) and baby is experiencing tachycardia, remove the source of heat and pack the mom with ice (armpits, lower back, lower abdomen, between thighs). Give appropriate herbs or meds for fever. I've seen this technique normalize a baby's heartbeat in 20 minutes.

Julila Joubert, NC

Soothing Pack

Apply a warm, wet towel to the woman's entire crotch area between contractions to soothe her and help her rest and relax.

Naolí Vinaver, Veracruz, Mexico

Perineal Massage Oil

Vitamin E/tochopherol is much better for perineal massage than olive oil because of its inherent absorption properties. It stays within the tissue for a longer amount of time to maintain elasticity, not just lubricity.

Renee, AOL

(Preventing Porlonged Labor, cont'd)

until the mother is approaching second stage and is one reason for her not feeling a pushing urge. She may say that she has supra-pubic pain while pushing. While you are certain that she is not completely dilated, or has a cervical lip, it will be the baby's elbow making pushing painful. Have the mother put counterpressure against the area while she bears down. She will know just how much pressure to use, as it is difficult for the attendant to gauge. When the baby delivers, check for a hand. If it is there, grasp it firmly, pulling it straight out while pressing firmly against the mother's perineum. This will facilitate delivery, while avoiding severe labial and vaginal tears.

Thoroughly familiarizing yourself with a variety of circumstances that could lead to prolonged labor not only helps you diagnose a condition when it presents but may make it possible to avoid transport to the hospital. Once we get beyond the standard pronouncement that there is failure to progress, we can take deliberate steps to facilitate a safe, successful delivery without medical intervention.

Twins: A Very Special Occurrence

by Valerie El Halta

SOMETHING ABOUT THE word "twin" seems to inspire an immediate anxiety attack in all concerned: mother, father, grandmother, midwife, and especially obstetrician. Medical literature abounds with information on multiple gestation and the inherent risks to the mother and her babies. Twins are generally viewed as pathology, and very little is written about the possibilities of achieving an optimum outcome. I do not consider "twinning" to be an anomaly, but a very special occurrence that deserves careful management to ensure safety for both mother and babies. Indeed, there is no reason the mother of twins cannot expect to deliver healthy full-term infants when she is properly educated, has a high level of responsibility and receives excellent prenatal care.

It is not my intent to either advocate or oppose the idea that the management of multiple pregnancies is beyond the scope of midwifery practice, or that out-of-hospital delivery of multiples should be considered. It is, however, my opinion that if one undertakes the practice of midwifery, one should be knowledgeable about all possible "variations of normal" that may—and are likely to—occur.

In fact, the first twins birth I attended caught me by surprise. The mother, new to my area, came to me in the second trimester. As I recorded her fundal height and found it to be above dates, I referred to her previous records and found she had equal measurements for dates with her first baby. Her son had weighed 10 pounds at birth, so I accepted the disparity as normal for her. At term, her fundus measured 44 centimeters. If I had been looking for twins, I probably would have discovered them, but because I assumed she was going to have another "whopper," I simply missed the signs. Her labor progressed smoothly and rapidly to second stage, when she pushed once and delivered a beautiful, small, baby girl into my hands. I immediately listened for another heartbeat and discovered a second baby, ready to be born. We were fortunate we had no complications, as the girls were identical (monozygotic babies have a greater likelihood of fetal anomalies and are at risk for developing twin-to-twin transfusion). Both babies weighed a little more than 5 pounds and were perfectly healthy. (A photograph of Robin and Sarah, peeking over their mother's shoulder while she is nursing them, is in Elizabeth Noble's book, *Having Twins*.)

Since then, I have been privileged to assist at the births of 27 sets of twins. (As I write, I am waiting for number 28.) Most of the deliveries have gone smoothly, some have been surprises, some have been carefully planned, but not all of them have had

(Continued on next page)

perfect outcomes. One second twin developed cerebral palsy as a result of a prolapsed cord. One baby girl, the first-born of identical twins, suffered a cardiac arrest in my arms at 1 1/2 hours postpartum. She was resuscitated and transported to the hospital, where she died of an undetermined anomaly at three weeks of age. Only once have I had to transport a mother to the hospital for a cesarean delivery of the second twin. This baby presented with her hand, face and cord! I shoved the baby back up the birth canal as high as I could, and transported them to the hospital. The surgeon had a hard time finding the baby, but fortunately she was delivered in great condition.

If you decide to take on the responsibility of assisting at the birth of twins, you must know there are risks involved. However, there is an element of risk in all birth, so my advice is: Learn all that you can, get as much experience as possible and proceed as your heart dictates. It is also important to understand that the new parents' needs will be much greater as they embark upon the awesome task of caring for two babies at once. Be prepared to assist them with concerns and to help them find competent support during the early weeks. Recognition of the reality of the "fourth trimester" is vitally important.

Prenatal preparation

"Super nutrition" is vital in assuring the health and well-being of both mother and babies. Many of the factors that place multiple pregnancies at risk may be virtually eliminated when the mother is adequately nourished, and this means "eating for three." The mother of twins is more at risk of developing preeclampsia due to the added stress upon her body. Yet, based on many years of experience with women of all risk categories, I am convinced this condition need never develop when adequate amounts of protein are consumed. Other conditions, such as anemia, varicosities, placental insufficiency, prematurity, hemorrhage, uterine dysfunction and uterine atony, are all hallmarks of a multiple gestation that are to be expected, according to obstetric literature. However, I believe these conditions may be completely preventable as well.

Consider Jane's case history, for example. Jane, 36, was pregnant for the first time. She had opted for career instead of family so was thrilled about the pregnancy and felt doubly blessed when her obstetrician announced she was having twins. However, Jane's joy was quickly overshadowed by his ominous predictions: probable spontaneous abortion before four months; a great likelihood that one or both babies may have chromosomal abnormalities. He recommended Jane undergo an amniocentesis due to her age.

After the test results revealed the babies were developing normally, Jane told me his next pronouncements, in rapid succession, were: she would surely develop preeclampsia; her babies would be born very prematurely (because twins are always premature due to overdistention of the uterus!); she would be scheduled for cesarean section at 37 weeks (to make sure they were born prematurely?). The obstetrician also told Jane she was not to gain more than 25 pounds. That was the extent of his advice, except for prescribing vitamins and telling her to quit her job.

Needless to say, Jane sought other care alternatives and eventually chose me to be her midwife.

I met Jane when she was about 16 weeks pregnant. After listening to her story, and calming her down, I told her there was no reason for a cesarean section just because she was carrying twins. If she developed complications that prohibited the possibility of a vaginal birth, we would transfer her to a hospital—as with any pregnancy. However, her pelvis was more than adequate, and she had no other preexisting negative health factors. I emphasized the importance of excellent nutrition, like I always do. I told Jane she would be expected to gain at least 50 pounds during the course of her pregnancy. After all, it takes work to carry two full-term babies, two healthy placentas, two amniotic sacs, and create some reserve weight for supporting the breastfeeding of two infants. Finally, I assured Jane if she would follow our program, there was every chance she would carry her babies safely to term.

Jane carefully studied all the information she could find and decided what I had advised her made sense. She felt very

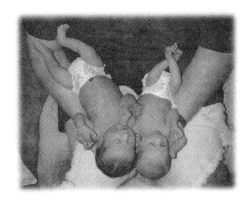

photo by Marilyn Nolt

strongly against having an elective cesarean section, as she felt this would lengthen the time of her recovery and hamper her ability to care for her newborns. This highly motivated mother kept all of her prenatal appointments, kept her food diary, ate 100 grams of protein daily, drank her water, walked a mile a day, and delivered two beautiful 7-pound babies at 38-1/2 weeks. The girl was in a military presentation; the boy went from a breech presentation to transverse to vertex. Not once did Jane show any signs of preeclampsia or suffer from any of the other maladies that so often plague mothers of multiples. She did gain her 50 pounds, most of which she had lost by her five-week checkup, and she successfully breastfed both of her children.

Important considerations

Why do so many multiple births happen prematurely? The medical theory is that not only does multiple pregnancy cause added stress on the maternal system but over-distention of the uterus causes premature contractions and labor. If that is so, then why do so many very large babies (more than 9 pounds) often go to term—or even become overdue? I have seen some very over-distended abdomens that not only carried large babies but a surplus of amniotic fluid as well, with fundal heights often measuring up to or greater than 45 centimeters. These women carried to term, some went overdue, and some had completely normal labors and deliveries. I sincerely believe most twins are born prematurely because they are suffering from starvation in utero, and thus come out early so that they can be fed!

Several important considerations should be noted when anticipating a twin delivery. These include: the mother's commitment to her nutrition and general health, the type of twins (fraternal,

(Continued on next page)

monozygotic, etc.), the placental attachment site, the position of the babies, and their growth and development. It must be noted that monozygotic twins have a greater likelihood of having fetal anomalies and are at risk for developing twin-to-twin transfusion. For this reason, I strongly advise clients to have at least three ultrasound examinations during the course of the pregnancy.

The first should be done at the time the multiple gestation is suspected or diagnosed. In my experience, this is usually between 16 weeks and 20 weeks. At this time, the gestational age and the type of twins expected are most easily diagnosed. We hope that even if only one placenta is seen (it is possible that two placentas have fused early in pregnancy), individual amniotic sacs will be identified. If both babies are within one amniotic sac, the delivery risk is very high, as the babies, and most important their umbilical cords, may become entangled. Many of the twins in this category do not survive pregnancy.

The second ultrasound should be done at about 30 weeks so that results can be compared with the first scans. At this time, problems such as intrauterine growth retardation (IUGR) may be diagnosed in one or both babies due to placental insufficiency, or any life-threatening anomalies in one or both babies can be identified so that preparations and plans can be made as to mode and place of delivery. An ultrasound at this time may also detect a discrepancy in size and estimated gestational age, which is possible when there is a separate conception date (rare) for the babies.

Also at the 30-week mark, if twin-to-twin transfusion is taking place, the babies will be remarkably dissimilar in size and weight, and the mother should be referred for high-risk care. In this case, the babies will be monitored closely and delivered as soon as they have reached sufficient maturity. Interestingly, the baby most at risk is the larger one, who has received a surplus of blood. This baby must be handled very delicately, as its internal organs have been stressed. Often, the suffused baby will require one or more exchange transfusions to first reduce and then supplant red blood cells. The smaller, anemic baby can simply be given extra blood.

It is wise to have at least one more ultrasound done as close to term as possible to verify the babies' presentation and position. Even with the most experienced hands, this information is often difficult to assess, as there are so many parts to feel!

A Study Outline on Twin Pregnancy, Labor and Delivery

by Valerie El Halta

THE FOLLOWING IS an outline for study and application purposes on twin pregnancy, labor and delivery.

I. Diagnosis
  A. History
    1. Type of twins
      a) Maternal more relevant
      b) Father responsible for monozygotic
    2. Frequency of occurrence
  B. Early symptoms
    1. All usual symptoms are usually escalated
      a) Nausea and vomiting, give more chance of hyperemesis gravidarum
      b) Probable obvious implantation bleeding (may misconstrue as a period)
      c) More fatigue and emotional fluctuation
  C. Fundal growth
    1. Question of size for dates, especially at 16-20 weeks
    2. Large increment of centimeters in short time (4 centimeters' growth in one week)
    3. Head size feels disproportionate to fundal height
  D. Excessive movement felt by mother
    1. Often missed by primaparas
    2. Multip will remark at how different this pregnancy feels
  E. "Too many parts"
  F. Auscultation of multiple, disparate fetal heart tones
  G. Ultrasound examination reveals twins

II. Hallmarks of Normal Pregnancy
  A. Increased nutritional needs
    1. Mother will be constantly hungry
    2. In late pregnancy, it will be difficult to eat due to enlarged uterus
      a) Encourage small, frequent, high-protein meals
      b) High-protein shake is well tolerated
    3. Will invariably have heartburn
  B. May have some back pain (sciatica), especially in last trimester
    1. Chiropractic treatments can help greatly
    2. Two babies in different positions throw pelvis out of line
  C. Excessive worry, nightmares and anxiety
    1. Due largely to hormonal surges
    2. Escalated by "friendly advice" from everyone
  D. Difficulty in sleeping
    1. Due to excessive fetal movement, other discomforts
    2. May be nature preparing mom for inevitable lack of sleep after birth!
  E. Hemorrhoids, irregular bowel movements
    1. Lots of pressure, no room, reduced activity, etc., all add to problem
    2. Encourage exercise, particularly walking
    3. Encourage high-fiber-food

ingestion and adequate water

III. Pregnancy Complications
- A. Anemia
    1. Usually difficult to raise hemoglobin above 11
    2. Do not oversupplement, sustain
- B. Hypertension, with or without other preeclampsia symptoms
    1. Due to extra stress on all maternal systems
    2. Suggest: calcium, 2 grams nightly
        a) Reduces hypertension
        b) Relieves muscle cramps
        c) Enhances sleep
- C. Prematurity or spontaneous abortion, early or late
    1. Greater incidence of fetal anomalies
    2. Predisposing health factors, age of mother, etc.
    3. Multiparous mothers may dilate prematurely due to excess weight and excess pressure that babies place on cervix
        a) Use of abdominal support device such as "prenatal cradle"
        b) Advise elevating foot of bed
    4. Parents may have to refrain from sexual activity late in pregnancy (last six weeks)
- D. Emotional and physical stress
    1. The mother needs an excellent support system both during and after pregnancy
        a) Much higher hormonal levels with twins
        b) B vitamins may assist emotional upheavals
    2. Mother needs extra rest. We require a two-hour afternoon rest with feet elevated
    3. Regular exercise is essential in providing oxygenation of muscles and relieving stress
        a) Swimming and walking are best
        b) Avoid jarring vertical movement such as impact aerobics

IV. Twin Labor
- A. Labor usually ensues at or about 38 weeks gestational age
    1. Note: Term for twins is 38 weeks!
    2. Gestation is actually escalated in multiples
        a) After 38 weeks there is usually some degree of IUGR symptoms, i.e., diminished subcutaneous fat stores, etc.
        b) Placentas show calcification
- B. Position and presentation
    1. Vertex, vertex
        a) Possible impaction (trying to come out at same time)
        b) Cord compression
        c) Failure to progress
    2. Breech, vertex
        a) Possible locked twins (baby A's chin locked with baby B's chin)
        b) Same complications as in all breech deliveries
    3. Breech, Breech
        a) Same complications as in all breeches
        b) Highest risk with footlings, either one or both, cord prolapse
    4. Vertex, Breech
        a) Most hospitals deliver breech by cesarean
        b) Risk of prolapse may be outweighed by accessibility to second baby
- C. Labor
    1. Longer prodromal stage
        a) Larger area of uterus to contract
        b) Babies may be vying for position
    2. Possible incoordinate uterine action
        a) In primaparas
        b) Larger uterine area
    3. Try to stop labor and rest mother
    4. Labor will ensue normally when restarting
    5. May be difficult to auscultate both fetal heart tones due to positions
        a) If difficult to hear second baby, try having mother lie on her side and go "behind baby A"
        b) Babies may have same heart rate
    6. Mother may have difficulty with nausea or vomiting due to pressure on diaphragm from distended uterus, especially during rise with contractions
    7. Important to keep mother well hydrated
    8. Watch blood pressure
    9. Possible for spontaneous rupture of membranes to occur with one sac only (and it may not be Baby A's)

V. Delivery of Twins
- A. Environment
    1. The birth room must be kept very warm, as it is expected that twins will usually be somewhat smaller and have less body fat than singletons, even at term
    2. Do not remove Baby A from the mother unless absolutely necessary
        a) The warmth of the mother's body will protect Baby A from hypthermia
        b) Baby A may nurse or nuzzle at mother's breast, stimulating resumption of contractions
        c) The weight of the baby (and babies) on mother's abdomen stimulates uterine contractions, escalating the return of labor, facilitating third stage and most importantly, prevents hemorrhage!
    3. Although it is important to have an adequate number of "helping hands" at the birth, be aware of the impact each person is having on the mother, her labor and her feelings of privacy.
    4. Too many observers can be detrimental should an emergency situation occur.
- B. Delivery of first twin
    1. Same delivery procedure as for singleton
    2. Clamp cord with hemostat designated for Baby A and sever
        a) If it is has been established that babies are fraternal, i.e., separate placentas observed by ultrasound, it is not necessary to prematurely separate cord
        b) Clamping cord important if babies are monozygotic due to possible transfusion
    3. Employ some means for identification of babies
        a) Twins will often look very much alike even if fraternal (unless different sex)
        b) We use a marking pen and

(Continued on next page)

Tips & Tricks

Nuchal Hand

Generally, if the pregnant woman is not obese, one can identify a nuchal hand up by the baby's face by palpating the mother's abdomen. If a pregnant mother has noticed her baby has hiccups, then probably her baby has been sucking his thumb, and that situation more times than not produces a nuchal hand at birth.

If you have a labor that is long or stalled with a large collar type of a cervix, this is usually either a cord that is holding the baby up or a nuchal hand.

A nuchal hand can keep a woman from going into labor, so if she is overdue by two weeks, check to see if you can palpate a hand from the outside and move it out of the way. On delivery, sometimes the hand can be pushed back up into the birth canal or extended out against the head of the baby. These procedures are only valid if you are expecting to deal with a nuchal hand; most of the time they are a surprise.

As far as preventing the perineum from tearing, the key of course is always controlled crowning, without or without a nuchal hand.

Cathy O'Bryant, CPM (E-News)

Enemas May Help Progress

A woman was 6 cm dilated, multiparous but not progressing, with a very loaded bowel. I gave her an enema (a rare thing for me), she had a bowel movement, and five minutes later ruptured membranes and delivered. A few weeks ago I was caring for a woman who was fully dilated with a full bowel. I was loath to give her an enema at that point, but did get her up onto a commode (hospital birth) to push. She had a small bowel movement, then got back on the bed and delivered. In the second instance I think it was a combination of the bowel movement and the position change that moved the baby down.

Kirsten Blacker (E-News)

Holding Back?

If a woman is holding back because she is afraid of passing a stool, suggest she sit on the toilet and push. Then offer her a bedpan AND some privacy.

Anon. (E-News)

write "A" on Baby A's foot.
C. Delivery of second twin
  1. Immediately assess position of second twin
  2. There is generally a respite from contractions as the uterus reforms around the reduced interuterine mass
  3. Be prepared to optimize position by external or internal version (or both)
     a) If baby is oblique, push head into delivery position
     b) If baby is "folded" (feet and hands) grasp feet and begin breech extraction
        (1) Version is dangerous and difficult once contractions resume
        (2) Baby B has great range of motion once Baby A is delivered
     c) Immediately and continuously take fetal heart tones
  4. Once Baby B is in an optimal position, it is wise to rupture membranes and stimulate contractions, to assure safe and timely delivery of Baby B
     a) Baby A at breast will stimulate return of contractions
     b) If Baby A is not cooperative, use manual stimulation
  5. It is not unusual for Baby B to be slower to respond than Baby A even if she has not had any apparent signs of distress
     a) Handle baby gently (as always)
     b) Be prepared to assist or resuscitate as necessary
  6. There is no need to hasten cord separation of Baby B

VI. Third Stage
A. Maintain strict observance of third stage protocol
  1. Be careful to not cause hemorrhage by excessive handling of the uterus
  2. Time beginning of third-stage after delivery of second twin
B. Watch for excessive bleeding
  1. One placenta may separate before delivery is complete
  2. A higher risk of abruption exists with the second twin
C. Both placentas usually deliver together even if fraternal twins
D. Examine placentas carefully
  1. There is a higher incidence of retained membranes
  2. It may be possible to detect evidence of placental fusion
  3. Look for crossing of blood vessels from one side of the placenta to the other
     a) Evidence of "identical" twins
     b) Look for any signs of fetal transfusion between babies
E. Watch for signs of sub-involution, such as a "boggy" uterus
  1. Fundal massage is indicated due to lack of uterine contractility after hyper-distension
  2. If hemorrhaging occurs, appropriate use of oxytoxics is indicated, as directed by physician

VII. Immediate Postpartum
A. Watch for signs of shock
  1. There has been a greater than usual loss of body weight for mother
  2. She may appear or feel as though she has lost too much blood, even when scant
B. Treat prophylactically
  1. Keep mother supine and elevate lower extremities
  2. Keep mother and babies warm
  3. Offer sweetened fruit juice or other high fructose beverages, as tolerated
C. Be prepared to stay with mother and baby for at least 12 hours postpartum
  1. It may take babies somewhat longer than normal to stabilize
  2. Mother needs to be watched for any signs of postpartum eclampsia
     a) More common after twins due to rapid changes in circulation, excessive fluid retention, etc.
     b) There is more necessity for immediate diuresis, yet slower kidney function
  3. Mother may be overwhelmed by reality of two babies

Natural Alternatives to Induction

by Marnie Ko ©1998

BABIES COME ON their own time according to their own timetable. In fact, it is now established that it is the baby in utero that stimulates the mother's body and hormones to initiate labor, not the mother, as was once thought. Due dates must be seen as a guide to an approximate time frame that the average pregnancy will last. Most pregnancies are not "average," and women can have their babies during the period between 36 to 38 weeks and 40 to 43 weeks and still be safe and within normal range. This should be reiterated strongly, as it is often tempting to want the baby to come much earlier than the baby is ready.

If it is established that the placenta is not doing well, a term woman is faring poorly in the last weeks of pregnancy, or issues arise as to safety and health of the mother or fetus, there are methods to gently and safely encourage labor without artificial induction.

It will benefit midwives, doulas and others in the birth field to have a ready reference guide to natural alternatives to artificial induction for instances when a woman is sure of her dates and waiting for the baby to come naturally is not feasible.

Artificial Induction

Doctors too commonly begin pressuring women to undergo induction. Induction carries with it negative implications including increased risk of complications, increased risk of infection (from invasive methods), fetal distress, greatly increased pain with contractions, a need for drugs that adversely affect both mother and infant, hypertonus of the uterus and fetal brachycardia. Induction is usually done with oxytocin infusion via intravenous or by vaginal prostaglandin followed by oxytocin, if required. There are worries that induction can cause more cases of failure to progress and increase the need for an emergency cesarean section.

There are a variety of ways that induction is accomplished—breaking the waters, mechanically stripping the membranes, and employing pharmacologic methods such as Pitocin or Syntocin drip via IV or the application of Pitocin intracervically or intravaginally. Pitocin is synthetic oxytocin, a pituitary hormone occurring naturally in the body that causes contractions of the uterus. Oxytocin is released by a woman's pituitary gland during labor, during sexual excitement and orgasm, and during breastfeeding. Oxytocin is used most often to induce labor, but it has an antidiuretic effect and like all methods of induction carries risks and complications.

Prostaglandin gel is also used regularly by medical professionals to induce labor, and it is applied to the cervix to cause it to dilate.

Before considering artificial induction, women may choose to investigate natural, non-invasive methods of encouraging labor when 40 to 43 weeks pregnant.

Sexual Activity

The simple act of lovemaking before or during labor facilitates a quicker birth and can trigger the onset of labor. When a woman is sexually stimulated, oxytocin flows through her system, causing her uterus to contract, either in the form of orgasms or labor contractions.

Lovemaking is without the negative consequences of synthetic Pitocin, but because of increased risk of infection it should not be undertaken if the waters have broken.

In addition, lovemaking provides naturally what prostaglandin gel tries to achieve artificially. And it is a pleasurable sensation as well. Intercourse deposits semen against the cervix of the woman, which works to soften the cervix, lengthen the pelvic ligaments and allow the baby's head to pass through with ease.

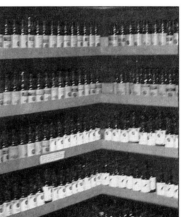

Prostaglandin inserts given in the hospital contain relaxin, the male seminal fluid responsible for these marvelous effects on the cervix, but the source of this synthetic relaxin is pig semen. Not only is this quite unappealing to most normal women, the benefits of relaxin are greatest when ingested orally, 10 times greater than if applied topically. Thus, oral sex with a spouse, with human relaxin, as part of lovemaking in late pregnancy or at term, has the added benefit of quickly providing effective encouragement to labor. And it isn't derived from pigs.

Blue and Black Cohosh

Blue cohosh is a powerful herb that regulates labor and increases the effectiveness of contractions. It is used to bring on active labor and regular contractions. Caulophyllum, another name for this herb, is very helpful for weak and irregular contractions. It relieves muscle spasms and stimulates uterine contractions. Its chemical and nutrient content includes calcium, coulosaponin, folic acid, gum, inositol, iron, leontin, magnesium, methylcystine, pantothenic acid, phosphoric acid, phosphorus, potassium, salts, silicon, starch, vitamin B-3 and vitamin E. It should not be used during the first two trimesters of pregnancy. Its other uses have included aiding the treatment of memory problems, menstrual disorders and disorders of the nervous system.

Black cohosh, or cimicifuga, is an herb that encourages regular, effective contractions and eases mothers' anxiety, worry and trepidation about labor. Its chemical and nutrient content includes

(Continued on next page)

actaeine, cimicifuin, estrogenic substances, isoferulic acid, oleic acid, palmitic acid, pantothenic acid, phosphorus, racemosin, tannins, triterpenes and vitamin A. Cimicifuga is also helpful for reducing blood pressure and cholesterol levels and decreasing mucous production. It relieves symptoms of menopause, including hot flashes and irregular bleeding, and eases menstrual cramps.

Using blue and black cohosh in combination is an extremely effective method of encouraging labor in the term woman when her baby is ready to come. Because this is one of the most aggressive means of starting labor, it is wise to consider receiving input and guidance from an experienced homeopath. Blue and black cohosh should not be tried prior to 39 weeks and then used only when a woman is sure of her dates.

Blue and black cohosh can be found in either pellet or liquid tincture form. Both are effective, and it is not necessary to find them both in the same form. If one is available in pellet and one in tincture, these two can be combined for the same results. One dose of small pellets that are the size of coarse salt is about five pellets. One dose of small pellets that are the size of peppercorns requires only three pellets. In liquid form, a dose is typically 10 to 20 drops in a teaspoon of water.

To encourage labor, blue and black cohosh can be taken in alternating doses, one herb each time, 30 minutes to an hour apart. A woman at 40 weeks may decide to start treatment slowly, with an hour between doses, while a woman nearing 42 weeks may wish to be more aggressive and leave only 30 minutes between doses. It is not advisable to take more than six to 10 doses in one day, with a complete stop of treatment the next day, and resuming treatment on the third day.

If there is no result after two full days of treatment, it would be safe to assume that the baby is not yet ready and needs more time in utero, as these herbs are extremely effective in safely encouraging labor, without side effects, when the baby and mother are ready.

Achyranthes

Achyranthis bidentatae is the botanical name of this herb, which has long been used in China for inducing labor. Its common name is achyranthes root or cyathula root, and it resembles small, pale, colored wood cylinders about 4 millimeters in diameter.

Achyranthes belongs to the family of *Amaranthaceae*, with about 850 species in 65 genera widely distributed in temperate and tropical regions. Many species of the family are intimately associated with humans as potherbs, as sources of edible seed and as troublesome weeds. Some are cultivated for their attractive flowers.

Achyranthes can be used in two ways to initiate labor. One-half to 1 ounce can be boiled and drunk as a tea, which will take between six hours to two days to produce an effect in most women. It can also be used internally by tying a thread around one piece of the root, inserting it vaginally, and pulling it out once contractions begin. Estimated time for this effect is a few hours to 24 hours.

The use of this root in childbirth is unfamiliar to many practitioners. However, a skilled and knowledgeable doctor trained in traditional Chinese medicine can provide guidance for the use of this herb for the purpose of beginning labor. It originates in China, Indonesia, Indo-China, Sri Lanka and Malaysia, and its Chinese name in English is Niu Xi.

Its many other uses include promoting circulation, dissolving clots, as an emmenagogue, and as a tonic to liver and kidneys.

Acupressure

Acupressure is another effective and safe method for inducing labor without the side effects of artificial induction. Acupressure for childbirth works by stimulating points of the body corresponding with the uterus to stimulate contractions. This is not the same as acupuncture, which uses needles inserted into the skin to achieve healing, as acupressure is simply pressure applied to certain points of the body for healing results.

If considering this method, it is wise to consult with a doctor of acupuncture and have him find the proper pressure points on the body. A woman might ask him to mark these points with a permanent felt marker so that when she is at home she can apply pressure to the points herself. One point of particular use is on the inside of the lower leg, between the two bones in that area, about 3-1/2 finger widths up from the ankle bone.

An additional point is found between the thumb and index finger. It can be pinpointed by finding the point just where the two bones of these fingers meet. Again, it is best to have these points marked by a doctor of acupuncture to be sure they are pressured accurately. These points are stimulated by the application of steady

(Continued on next page)

Tips & Tricks

Love the Baby Out

The best way to induce naturally for most mothers is to have sex! After intercourse the woman should try to keep the semen around her cervix for as long as is comfortable. Semen contains the wonderful natural prostaglandins that help ripen the cervix. Orgasm also releases hormones that promote uterine activity.

If a woman is not able to have intercourse, nipple stimulation is also useful. If women are birthing in hospital settings, privacy should be allowed for these activities.

Amanda Gear, Australia (E-News)

Visualize the Baby Out!

In private meditation or with someone helping you, do guided visualization, go deep within and listen, asking your baby why s/he has not yet decided to go through the birth process. It is the baby who initiates labor. Unlimited answers are possible and might include: fear of the birth process (yours or the baby's); aversion to one or more participants or location planned for the birth; or your feelings of lack of readiness for parenthood. (It may seem as if the answer is coming from your imagination, but your imagination is an important part of your mind.) Then listen for any possible solutions that may be offered.

Donna Worden-Wonder (E-News)

pressure for 10 minutes at a time or by vigorous rubbing of the spot,

If acupressure is used, it is best tried alone and not in conjunction with homeopathy, as these are both powerful remedies that work in different ways on the body. Acupressure, however, is not as much of an issue with homeopathics as is acupuncture, which can interfere with the action of homeopathics if taken in conjunction. Acupressure on the points to stimulate the uterus as described above can be uncomfortable because they are very sensitive and tender during pregnancy. If it does cause discomfort, it means the proper spot has been found.

An additional, painless acupressure method involves no active pressure applied, which may be an option that appeals to some pregnant women. This must be undertaken under the care of an acupuncturist, and some of them will not charge, or will charge a very nominal fee for this. It involves tiny steel balls the size of a grain of salt being placed in the ear, usually on three spots in the ear that stimulate the uterus to contract.

These balls are anchored with very sticky round pieces of tape and cannot be seen unless someone is specifically looking for them. They are to be taken out once active labor is accomplished (so that they do not increase the strength of contractions unnecessarily). A special instrument is used to pinpoint the proper locations in the ear to place the balls, and the benefits of this method are that it is fast, painless, inexpensive and has no side effects. It also does not require anything of the pregnant woman once they are in place, other than to remember to remove them once they take effect.

Castor Oil

Castor oil is no longer a remedy that desperate pregnant women must employ to initiate labor. Castor oil contains some of the essential fatty acids that are used by the human body to create prostaglandins. Not only does it cause horrific cramps, nausea, vomiting, and spastic uterine contractions in some women, it is downright unpleasant, even if disguised in an orange juice "cocktail."

It works to stimulate labor by irritating the intestine into contractions, which create a corresponding reflex contraction in the uterine muscles. If the woman is ready to give birth and the cervix is ripe (soft and beginning to dilate), these contractions can become uterine contractions resulting in labor. There is, however, no guarantee. The worry and reluctance to use castor oil stem from a relative lack of knowledge of exactly how it affects mother and baby, and what level of prostaglandins are actually contained in it. Castor oil can cause uncontrolled uterine activity; spasmodic, painful contractions; and hyperstimulation of the uterus, which can result in fetal distress, the passage of meconium and increased risk of intervention. It is not recommended.

Senna Tea

An alternative to castor oil—which has a questionable, undetermined role in stimulating the bowels, in turn stimulating the uterus—is senna tea. Senna tea has a gentle laxative effect that stimulates the sympathetic contraction of the uterus as well as the bowel, since they are both made of a type of muscle tissue called smooth muscle. This stimulation is often enough to begin labor in a woman who is term or past 40 weeks. Senna is purchased dried in leaf form and steeped in boiling water to make tea. It is typically steeped for half an hour, and can be steeped for up to two hours, and a dose may be half a cup to one cup. This is entirely dependent on how quickly the woman wants to progress and if she wants to start slowly and judge the effects in addition to the suggestions she receives from her health care provider, if applicable.

Goldenseal

Goldenseal is a potent herb akin to an herbal antibiotic or a powerful disinfectant. Conflicting information on the use of goldenseal during pregnancy has created debate on its use for childbirth. It contains hydrastine, which causes uterine contractions if taken in large quantities, but it is unclear what a large quantity is and what dose is necessary to be effective. Because it contains high amounts of very potent alkaloids in addition to a strong antibiotic called berberine, it should be discussed with a knowledgeable herbalist before being used in childbirth.

(Continued on next page)

Tips & Tricks

Remedy the Baby Out
Homeopathic remedies pulsatilla 1m and caulophyllum 200c are often prescribed for natural induction. It may be necessary to treat mental blockages also.
Glenis (E-News)

Walk the Baby Out
To bring on labor try curb walking. I know it sounds funny, but I really believe it helps. Walk along a curb, one foot up on the curb and one in the gutter, then turn around and go the other way.
Calista (E-News)

Breastpump the Baby Out
At 11 days late, I used my double electric breast pump for 10 minutes on and 10 minutes off, over and over again for a four-hour period (I discarded the tiny bit of colostrum collected). Also at each 10-minute break, I swished and swallowed a blue and black cohosh concoction (three squirts each of high quality tincture). This was not fun but better than the alternative. That evening I had cramping but not contractions. I repeated it the next day, and after two hours contractions began. After that, the entire labor was 90 minutes start to finish, but that's another story!
Wendy Jones (E-News)

Why Induce?
I know some advocate induction near the due date because they think it will avoid problems with big babies, but the rate of fetal growth slows down near term. The average baby will gain no more than 4 to 8 ounces during that additional two-week period. This quarter to half-pound gain is hardly likely to significantly affect the birth outcome.
Gail Hart (E-News)

Commercial Products

NF Formulas (a Portland, Oregon, company) makes a homeopathic product called Matrigin. It contains caulophyllum (blue cohosh), arnica (for bruising and trauma), cimicifuga (black cohosh), pulsatilla and gelsemium. Dolisos makes a similar product called Childbirth Combo. Pulsatilla is a homeopathic often used for intermittent contractions that do not establish into consistent labor. Gelsemium, effective in ripening the cervix, is used to begin labor and is especially indicated when there is a conscious or subconscious fear of birth.

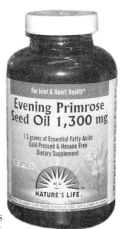

This remedy is also used as a preventative measure for women who go past their due date.

Pulsatilla

Pulsatilla is a common remedy used in labor. It can ease the pains of pre-labor (also called false labor) if taken in 200c potency every two hours for a maximum of three doses. If a woman is ready for labor, her contractions will become consistent and more powerful; if she is not ready, the contractions will cease.

Evening Primrose Oil

Evening primrose oil aids the ripening or softening of the cervix, preparing it to dilate. It softens the cervical tissue, which is very useful, when there is scar tissue from a previous surgery, abortion or damage from contraceptives (such as IUDs). It can be taken orally in a dose of three to six capsules per day and, like male seminal fluid, helps lengthen the pelvic ligaments so that the baby's head can engage properly in the pelvis. This will aid the process of dilation and can contribute to a quicker, less painful birth.

Using evening primrose oil may be a wise course of action for women who have had previous c-sections for failure to progress or who have labor that starts and stops. Evening primrose oil should not be taken sooner than the 36th week of pregnancy, and one to two capsules can also be used as a vaginal suppository, inserted at bedtime for increased effectiveness.

Aromatherapy

Certain aromatherapy essential oils can help activate labor and are typically applied through massage to the abdomen. The essential oils most effective for uterine stimulation are lemon, clarysage and fennel. Some practitioners will create a blend of lemon and clarysage or other oils for aid in childbirth. It is best to buy the essence of the oil and add it to a massage oil such as olive oil, jojoba oil, apricot, grapeseed (which is the easiest, most non-greasy oil to clean from the skin), and avocado oil, rather than buy it pre-prepared. It is less expensive and more pure when prepared by yourself.

Essential oil treatment can be through inhalation—inhaling the essence on a cloth or right from the bottle. It can also be diluted and added to a carrier oil, as listed above, in the ratio of three drops essential oil to one cup of carrier oil.

Essential oils are not considered to be drugs, but to be cosmetics that are applied topically or as dietary supplements that are regulated as "foods." Other oils worth researching for their aids in encouraging labor include rosemary, rose, myrrh, basil, chamomile, hyssop, juniper, lavender and marjoram. Consult an experienced aromatherapist for more information.

Motherwort

Motherwort is a bitter herb that is used to treat menstrual disorders when periods are inconsistent or stopped, and it is also highly effective as a uterine stimulant to encourage labor. It is commonly found in herbal combinations to regulate menstrual periods. Dosage is commonly 10 to 30 grams and can be found in leaves and also prepared in capsule form.

Wild Ginger

Wild ginger is used to improve circulation, aid digestion, eliminate flatulence and regulate periods. Many cultures use it steeped in tea to fight colds and flu. The Porno Indian people of California quite commonly drank it as tea just before menstruation to have lighter blood flow and less cramping. In doses of two to five grams, and under the care of a herbalist, it can be used to encourage labor at term.

Pennyroyal

Pennyroyal is an essential oil commonly used to regulate menstrual periods, rid the body of toxins through sweating and for colds and flu. It is often infused as tea, applied externally as a bug repellent or taken in capsules for a variety of conditions

Pennyroyal is a powerful essential oil in diluted form and should never be ingested in early pregnancy because of its abortive effect on the developing fetus, or the great risk of fetal damage. Under

(Continued on next page)

> ### Tips & Tricks
> **Emergen-C and Bleeding**
>
> While Emergen-C is indeed a great electrolyte booster, the high content of vitamin C can cause excessive bleeding after birth, surgery, dental work or other "bleeding potential" events. High doses of vitamin C can promote anti-coagulation. Caution should be exercised when employing this powder during labor. Dr. Andrew Weil (*Spontaneous Healing*) cautions against high doses of vitamin C before surgery. While childbirth isn't surgery, one bleeds naturally.
>
> Since we are all concerned that mothers do not bleed more than necessary, the use of regular strength "Emergen-C" during childbirth is not a good idea. Diluting it in twice or three times the water called for in the package directions may be a more appropriate solution than using it full strength. This dilution would then reduce the total Vitamin C intake accordingly.
> For a better option, try this:
>
> "Labor Aid" Mix
> 1 qt. water
> 1/3 c. honey
> 1/3 c. juice from a real lemon
> 1/2 t. salt
> 1/4 t. baking soda
> 2 crushed calcium tablets
>
> Serve cold or freeze into small ice cubes.
> *Kim Mosny, CPM (E-News)*

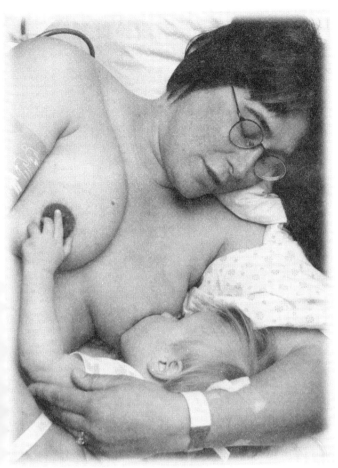

photo by Patti Ramos

supervision and with guidance, pennyroyal in a dosage of three to six grains may be an option in encouraging labor at term.

Safflower

Also known as *Carthamus tinctorius*, the Chinese name is Hong Hua. This remedy uses flowers from the safflower and promotes circulation, dissolves clots, acts as an emmenagogue and an astringent, and is used for postnatal abdominal pain, clots or seepage of blood in the abdominal region, traumatic injuries and stiffness in pain or joints. The recommended dose is two to five grams, and it can be used to encourage a reluctant labor at term.

Oxytocin Production

There are a variety of ways to increase the production of oxytocin. Nipple stimulation is one way to accomplish this, and such methods as breastfeeding a younger child, applying a warm towel to both breasts for five minutes, or massaging one nipple for 10 minutes have been shown to induce adequate uterine contractions in 20 minutes or less.

Walking is an activity that naturally releases oxytocin, as does exercise and sexual activity, as previously discussed.

Different things work for different pregnancies, and any woman who is reaching term and feeling anxious about birth or experiencing no obvious signs of physical readiness for birth should first consider her emotional state of mind and her physical environment. Is she relaxed? Does she feel safe? Are there any issues standing in the way of birth? Is her relationship with her spouse secure and strong? Is she comfortable with her birth plans? Is she fully aware of her options in birth and has she chosen a birth environment that is right for her? Is everything ready for the baby, and is she ready to become a mother? Once these emotional issues are looked at and resolved, it may be that a woman wishes to encourage labor by trying one or more of these suggestions.

In conclusion, there are a number of alternatives available to the often overused and very painful artificial induction. Many of these are listed here with the purpose of inspiring a woman to take responsibility for her birth and investigate these suggestions, choosing the course of action she feels most appropriate for her situation. In no way is any particular remedy or idea an endorsement of any or all methods. Rather, it is a starting point for a woman who is ready to be proactive when it comes to her health and her baby but who has previously been unable to find information on this subject.

As her caregiver, you can make this information available to her so that she can research, become informed and discuss these alternatives carefully.

It is important to emphasize to all caregivers of pregnant women that all of labor and birth are in the control of the birthing mother's thoughts and mind. She must be ready emotionally, spiritually and psychologically to give birth before her body will prepare physically for the hard and rewarding work ahead.

Tips & Tricks

Foot Bath

I love a hot water foot soak to get rid of a headache. We had a client who had a bout of flu at the time labor began, and the foot soak rid her of her headache so that she could concentrate on her labor.

Brenda Shea, LDEM, OR

Exhaustion and Sleep

I often joke with a first-time mother who is preoccupied with watching the clock that no woman has ever missed her birth by sleeping through it. It is important that the mother be encouraged to rest and sleep as much as possible in very early labor. If exhaustion has occurred, labor will slow down, and inertia and constriction rings may lead to operative intervention. The risk of maternal hemorrhage increases, as well as the possibility of subinvolution with excessive bleeding and postpartum infection.

Valeria El Halta, CPM (E-News)

Cervical Scarring

I have been a labor and delivery nurse for years and am an aspiring midwife. I have found that oftentimes cervical procedures such as laser surgery produce tough scarring that takes a bit longer to get going, but once the scarring has been broken up with a little digital manipulation, the cervix has the potential to open much more rapidly.

Becky (E-News)

"Good" Contraction

If a woman is having a hard time during labor, acknowledge it; remind her to do only one contraction at a time. Describe a hard contraction as a "good" one. When you make suggestions, tell her why the shower feels so good, why a walk will move things around, why a change of scene is good, why you're going to give her some privacy, why making deep sounds will open her up.

Linda McHale, CPM
Barbara Noble Schelling, CPM

Sterile Water Blocks for Back Pain in Labor

by Sharon Glass Jonquil, CNM

"My back! My back!" she screamed, clutching awkwardly at the sides of her little tummy while trying to relieve her back labor. Christy was a 19-year-old Caucasian gravid 3 para 2 at 35-36 weeks' gestation; she had spontaneously ruptured membranes (SROM) and began contracting at 5 o'clock in the morning. She arrived at the hospital six hours later, writhing in pain, with her supportive husband at her side. She was 4 centimeters dilated, 100 percent effaced, and her baby was at +2 station.

I had seen Christy a few days ago in the hospital to rule out SROM, and I had also seen her a couple of times in the clinic. She was a small, thin woman, with a difficult social history—her mother had put her up for adoption at birth, then changed her mind and kept her. They were currently estranged. Christy cut her one-pack-a-day smoking habit to two to three cigarettes a day during pregnancy, and her asthma was kept under control with Ventolin. An upper respiratory infection was treated with penicillin. She gained a total of 23 pounds during her pregnancy.

We breathed together while I helped her calm down and center herself for the work of labor. I offered her sterile water blocks (or papules) for her back pain. In theory, the blocks work because hyperstimulation of a skin area can affect perception of visceral pain. Nerves that supply the cervix and uterus end in skin in the lower back area and may cause "referred" pain. I explained it would involve four shots over her sacral area that would burn severely for 20 seconds to one minute, and then her back pain would be relieved for 45 minutes to three hours. She agreed to have the procedure done.

The labor nurse and I positioned ourselves with two tuberculin syringes filled with sterile water. Christy remained curled on her side during the procedure. After marking the four locations lightly with a pen and swabbing the area with alcohol, we warned her and simultaneously injected 0.15 cc subdermal into each of the two lower spots and then quickly the two upper areas. She shouted, "That hurts worse than the contractions!" We assured her the pain would pass promptly.

When her next contraction came three minutes later, a look of relief and surprise flashed over her face. The painful back labor was gone, as was the pain caused by the injection. Now she had only the intensity of regular labor contractions to deal with. We continued to work closely together. She requested a dose of IV medication. I gave her 1cc of Fentanyl, and she relaxed and coped beautifully with transition. At one point she remarked, "I forgive my mother everything." I asked for clarification: "You mean because she hurt like this to give you life?" "Yes!" she exclaimed. Soon she was bearing down, and we prepared for her son's birth. Slowly a little conehead emerged.

We softly gave Christy words of encouragement. Two nursery nurses stood by, ready to help if the baby had preterm problems. A third-year medical student was observing in the background with Christy's permission. The baby's head crowned and his shoulders slipped out. Christy pulled him up and out of her vagina and to her chest. She was

(Continued on next page)

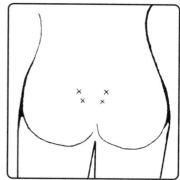

Illustration by Gert Welsh

Dear Gert Welsh,
I tried the intradermal water papules you spoke about at the Midwifery Today 1997 Orlando conference in September. WOW! WOW! WOW! I have never been so impressed with a trick as this one. I used it the other day on a 43-year-old gravid 3 para 2 who was having a lot of back discomfort. We had her husband doing back pressure until I suggested the water papules. She was 7 centimeters dilated at that point. The very next contraction after the injections changed her whole demeanor. She actually sat back in the rocking chair and said, "Wow! I don't even feel like I'm in labor anymore."

Every midwife, nurse and doctor should know how to do this one [technique].
Sara Liebling, CNM

Tips & Tricks

Holding Back?
If a woman is holding back because she is afraid of passing a stool, suggest she sit on the toilet and push. Then offer her a bedpan AND some privacy.
Anon. (E-News)

Ring of Fire
I try to prepare women for controlled pushing at the end by describing the "ring of fire" and saying it is a good thing to have because it means they haven't torn yet. I know that it helps moms be less afraid, to believe they can do it, and to cooperate at the critical time.
Cynthia Flynn, CNM, PhD (E-News)

worried—why was he so gray? "He's fine, just fine, watch him pink up," we reassured her. His muscle tone grew firm and his complexion bloomed pink. We gave him Apgars of 8 and 9. Daniel, the happy daddy, cut the cord with glee. Tony, their son, weighed five pounds, three ounces, and was 17 inches long. Christy's placenta delivered with ease, somewhat calcified even at this early gestation, perhaps because of her smoking.

Afterward I asked her about the injections and her back pain. She reiterated that they hurt "like an electric knife," but after the two minutes of pain she had complete relief from back labor for the rest of her labor, and she emphatically stated she would choose it again.

In the last months our practice has had experience with about 30 attempts using sterile water injections with 28 successes. The key is that it must truly be back labor, particularly caused by occiput posterior (OP) positioning of the baby.

Our midwifery practice is convinced that sterile water blocks for relief of back labor will revolutionize care for these women. It is easy to perform, it is safe for both mother and child, and it can be done in any setting. It may be repeated as needed. It requires only a tuberculin syringe, sterile water, knowledge of how to give subdermal intracutaneous injections, and a basic understanding of anatomy. How I wish I had learned about it years ago!

Birth Balls
by Joy Johnston, Midwife

DURING THE PAST couple of decades midwives around the world have actively sought ways to demedicalise childbirth and restore the birthing woman's authority over her body. Women are encouraged to be active in labour, choose their support people, use local warmth and touch rather than medical analgesia, use water for relaxation, and choose their place and positions for birth.

During the past years balls have bounced onto the birthing scene after having been used in other areas of health and fitness. The principles of good posture, muscle balance and stabilisation, gentle pelvic movement, and relaxation achieved by using fitness balls can be readily applied to the birthing woman. Balls also have the potential for relieving nervous tension, as they trigger memories of childhood play. The birth ball is easy to clean, can be used on the floor, in the shower, or on the bed, and provides a comfortable alternative seat or back support for a member of the birth team if the labouring woman isn't using it.

What Happens When a Labouring Woman sits on a Birth Ball?

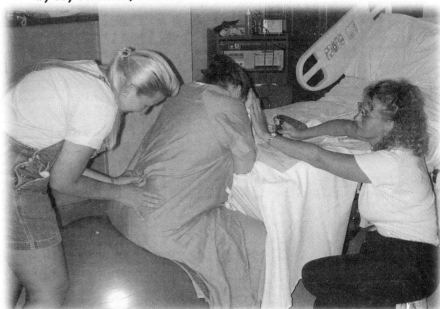

photo by Marilyn Nolt

- Her knees are apart, and there is no adductive muscle tension;
- Pressure on her entire sitting area is equalised, as opposed to the excessive pressures she might experience when she sits on a toilet or birthing stool;
- The woman's pelvic inlet is tilted forward in relation to her spine, which facilitates an occipito-anterior position of the fetal head;
- The dynamic nature of the supporting surface means any movement by the woman initiates a wave of corresponding movements;
- Pelvic tilting—both lateral and anterio-posterior—is made easy;
- Gentle exercise of the abdominal, back and pelvic floor muscles occurs without conscious control;
- It is easy to get up off the ball and return to it later.

Following are some comments I've heard from midwives who have attended women using birth balls for labour:

"A primip used the birth ball in the shower to rest on between contractions and to roll on during contractions. It worked well when her legs got too tired."

(Continued on next page)

"A lovely multip who had a history of quick labours sat on the ball in the shower with her husband hosing her. There was no pressure on the perineum. The baby was able to crown and the ball was pushed away for the birth of the rest of the body. I loved her delivery!"

"The ball provided a lot of comfort to a multip whose labor lasted just six hours. Labour progressed well and the mother loved it. The ball really opened her up and gave her some physical comfort."

"I used the ball for a multip in strong labour who needed to kneel but remain upright, so I put the ball on top of a bean bag against the bed. She stayed in this position until just before her birth. It was great because it didn't collapse and lose its form like bean bags do."

"A primip came to the hospital in early labour with mild contractions five to seven minutes apart. She sat on the ball while we completed admission, then she and her partner went for a long walk. Labour progressed well. She used the ball to rest on rather than a chair or the bed. She spent late first stage and most of second stage in the shower, either standing or on the ball. It was an active birth, and both parents were ecstatic."

"A multip had had a difficult first birth, and she was frightened by strong contractions and back pain. Sitting on the ball relieved back pain and the woman relaxed. Later when she stood in the shower, labour became very strong and she went into transition. The woman became anxious again and doubted her ability to continue. She then sat on the ball and felt relief. The woman soon said she felt the baby coming and she wanted to push."

"A homebirth primip had used the ball to sit on from about 38 weeks as well as in early labour. She progressed well to uncomplicated birthing."

There is no magic in using balls for birthing. As in the care of any woman, the skilled midwife is vigilant and advises the woman appropriately, seeking assistance when necessary. The birth balls enhance early labour by facilitating optimal fetal positioning in relation to the woman's pelvis and spine. They also provide comfort and relaxation and maintain a dynamic environment within the pelvic region, possibly avoiding slow progress for some women.

Birth balls are an exciting, new and inexpensive device for use in the maternity scene.

Tips & Tricks

Super Glue for HSV-II

The midwife I apprentice with suggests the use of "super glue" during delivery when a mother is infected with herpes. She applies the glue directly to the lesion, and it protects the infant from contact. She has yet to have an infant be affected by the virus, after more than fifteen years of practice.

Leighza (E-News)

Share With Your Community

One March, on a whim, I contacted the organizers of our local Earth Day festival and said "Breastfeeding is an environmental issue, right? Hundred dollar fetoscopes are non-invasive and more accurate than $15,000 electronic monitors, right?" Several similar remarks later, our local independent birth educators' organization was signed up to do an educational display table, at no charge, for the outdoor festival at a local park.

For the table, we made posters that identified our philosophy; one said "Natural Birth and Midwifery" and the other proclaimed "Breastfeeding and Earth-Friendly Parenting." We made phone calls across the country to every relevant 800 number we found. Merchants on the other end of our phone lines sent catalogs and discount coupons. We had information on cloth diapers, wooden toys, cloth menstrual products, birth-related books and products and much, much more. We distributed information about our local classes and other birth related services. One of our favorite "duties" was passing out the various brochures we had about babywearing devices to parents who were weary of pushing balky strollers through the park's sandy soil. We talked and made referrals until we were hoarse.

Start now to lay the ground work for participating in your community's Earth Day or other events. You will be glad you did, and so will those whose lives you touch.

Tricks of the Trade Circle, FL 1997

Grassroots Organizing

To organize a grassroots movement in support of midwifery and natural birth, use these four steps.

1. Identify people you know who are interested in supporting midwifery and natural birth; get them together in one place. The group will soon get the sense there is strength in numbers. Begin to recognize and get to know one another, talk and share ideas, hopes, dreams, commitments.

2. Identify a key person in the group who is a natural organizer, is dynamic, organized and is a good speaker. She will solidify the group and be its spokesperson.

3. Determine what strengths and talents each group member has: who is a good writer, who could organize a database, who excels at speaking. Then put them to work.

4. At every workshop or forum, circulate a form on which each attendee can write her name and address. Then reach out to them. Now the circle is widening, and strength is gained in numbers.

Clarebeth Kassel-Loprinzi, OR

Birth

Normalizing the Breech Delivery

by Valerie El Halta

During my 20-year career as a practicing midwife, I have often come under harsh criticism for continuing to attend what many consider to be "high-risk" deliveries. I have caught more than 20 sets of twins, assisted with more than 100 successful VBACs (vaginal birth after cesarean), and have caught more than 100 babies who happened to choose a breech position.

I remain adamant in my belief that these deliveries, while demanding great respect, do not necessarily portend greater risk to either mother or her baby. Of course, each situation needs to be carefully evaluated for inherent risks. However, I have seen many more high-risk situations develop in seemingly normal vertex births than I have yet to encounter in well-assessed and well-managed twin, VBAC or breech deliveries.

I am grateful for the numerous mothers and babies who have benefited by the technological advances in obstetrics and neonatology. Yet at the same time, I am appalled by the amount of empirical knowledge that has been cast aside for the sake of technical advancement.

Today, several competent midwifery schools offer a strong didactic program yet ignore the necessity for educating students in the technique of breech delivery, declaring that these deliveries pose such great risk they should never be attempted by the midwife. They seem to assume that by teaching this art, the midwife is given a sense of "permission" that would be inappropriate. I sincerely disagree with this philosophy, as I believe that the aspiring midwife should be schooled in every possible contingency of the birth process.

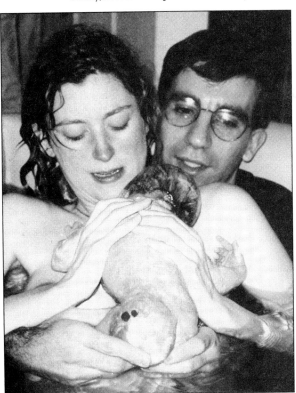

photo by Judith Halek

The day will come when a midwife encounters that "surprise" situation in which she finds herself powerless to act—much to the detriment of the mother and her baby, whom she is sworn to help. Walking into a labor at 3 a.m., 40 minutes away from the nearest hospital, and finding the baby out to its armpits affords no time to get out the books or to regret one's lack of knowledge!

"Oh, but that will never happen to me!" you may say. Don't count on it; it has happened to me! You will never harm the mother or baby by having an overabundance of knowledge and you will never regret having it.

The medical professional's reluctance to deliver the breech baby is well founded. Based upon their experience, this delivery is fraught with danger. How can we expect a physician to handle the unusual delivery when he has not been trained to allow the normal delivery?

(Continued on next page)

Tips & Tricks

Breech Issues

I believe a lot of breeches happen in second and subsequent pregnancies because the mother is carrying a 30-pound 2-year-old on her "bump" for the entire pregnancy. If the baby is breech, that weight on his head every day can predispose him to settle into the pelvis in that position. Warn the mother of a toddler not to use her pregnant belly as a platform for heavy objects of any kind. Dad can carry the 2-year-old more often, or she can use her hip as a support.

Gloria Lemay (E-News)

To turn a breech baby, some mothers find the slant board position uncomfortable and instead elect to choose a hands and knees position with their head and chest lowered close to the floor. Pillows are needed to be comfortable. Whatever the method, after a baby turns, spend a lot of time walking and squatting during Braxton Hicks contractions to encourage your baby to engage in the pelvis and minimize the chance of a return to a breech position.

Maryl Smith (E-News)

After the baby turns, continue to place music at the bottom of the abdomen to encourage the baby to stay head down. I have seen it work so many times that I routinely recommend "musical version" to anyone with a breech presentation.

Kathy Herron (E-News)

Nuchal Hand

Palpation may reveal a nuchal hand. A slow, guided delivery is important. I have seen a birth with nuchal hand happen without a tear. Hot compresses to stretch the perineum were used. Downward guidance was used to keep the woman from tearing upward.

Beth (E-News)

If you see a hand come with the head, or feel a hand when you feel for the cord, simply give the hand or fingers a little pinch and the baby will usually retract it.

R.H. (E-News)

Tips & Tricks

Breech With Extended Arms

I work in a high-volume maternity clinic in South America. For extended arms when the baby is breech, I have found the Lovset Maneuver works marvelously. It is safer, I understand, than sweeping the arms down manually with your fingers. This maneuver involves turning the baby 180 degrees, always keeping the back uppermost to sweep down the arm. It can be repeated to bring down the second arm. I refer you to Myles' midwifery text for a detailed description.

Lois Yoder, Paraguay, SA

Stand Up for Dystocia

When I was confronted with a classic case of shoulder dystocia, we tried the usual techniques to dislodge the baby. The shoulders were directly transverse, way up there and wedged. I couldn't get them to budge, and I was preparing for the next step—Wood's corkscrew—when I had a sudden inspiration: I asked the mom to stand up! The baby twisted and fell out; dad and I barely caught him! I guess the movement jiggled him loose and he came flying out. The head was born at 4:24, body at 4:31; the baby weighed 9 pounds, 2 ounces, with Apgars of 9 and 10.

Gail Hart, America Online

Cool It

I had a primip with an especially stubborn anterior lip. I used all the standard tricks with no success. She was begging me to "do something that will work." After telling her my intentions and receiving her permission, I put a piece of ice right up against the swollen anterior lip. I used four pieces in quick succession, holding each one on the lip and moving it from side to side until it melted. She said it felt good. Within four contractions the anterior lip was gone and she was ready to push.

I have used this trick many times since with great success. The lip just slips away. Women seem to like the cool feeling.

Dixie Story, NV

Rushing = Bleeding

Management of second stage can influence blood loss. Pushing before full dilation, coached pushing, fundal pressure and rushing the shoulders (delivering before full restitution and the second contraction after birth) can also increase bleeding and problems with the placenta.

Gail Hart (E-News)

Indeed, complications may ensue in the process of labor and delivery, and in no way do I wish to disallow them. Yet I believe that many of these complications may be avoided with competent knowledge of the mechanics of the breech labor and appropriate delivery technique.

Physiological Reasons for Breech Presentation

1. Prematurity
2. Placenta previa
3. Hydrocephalus
4. Multiparity
5. Hydramnios
6. Uterine abnormality
7. Tumors or fibroids
8. Multiple gestation

Other than these obvious physiological reasons for breech presentation, I believe the baby chooses the position that is most comfortable and that will guard him against oxygen deprivation. For example, I have delivered three breech babies who had complete knots in the cord. If they had been born vertex, they may have suffered hypoxia or been stillborn. Also, it is not unusual to find that the placenta, though not a previa, is somewhat low-lying (most often delivering Duncan), which leads me to wonder if the baby assumes the breech position to avoid the greater weight of his head pressing against the placental site, thereby reducing oxygen flow.

When considering a vaginal breech delivery, it is imperative the mother is emotionally stable, has a high degree of confidence in her body as well as in her midwife, and has a high degree of motivation. In attempting breech delivery, excellent communication and cooperation between the mother and her birth attendant are crucial. Allow extra time for a careful discussion with the parents so that they will know what to expect.

Complications of Breech Labor and Delivery

1. Greater incidence of cord prolapse, particularly with footlings
2. Pressure on the cord in first stage
3. Increased incidence of premature placental separation
4. Head entrapment due to pushing before, or misdiagnosis of, complete dilation
5. Injury to the head or neck
6. Increased danger of nerve damage if arms are swept up over the head

A Vaginal Breech Delivery Should Not Be Attempted Under the Following Conditions:

1. Suspected cephalopelvic disproportion (CPD)
2. Possibility of baby weighing more than 8 pounds or less than 5 pounds
3. Post-term infant (more than 40 weeks)
4. Preterm infant (earlier than 37 weeks)
5. Prior history of CPD or necessity for forceps delivery
6. Previous need for Pitocin induction or augmentation
7. Previous shoulder dystocia
8. Previous history of protracted or obstructed labor in first or second stage (except posterior)
9. Possible intrauterine growth retardation (IUGR)
10. Any evidence of fetal distress

Breech Scoring Index

When deciding the feasibility of attempting a breech delivery, the following index is of great help. However it remains paramount that the midwife use her own judgment

(Continued on next page)

as well. Never attempt a delivery for which you have neither the skill nor the experience. Even when you have determined that there are no predisposing factors against the delivery, if your heart shouts "No!" don't do it!

This assessment is designed to be made at the onset of labor. A client would be scored as follows: a multip (score 2) with a baby who weighs between 7 pounds and 8 pounds (score 1), at station -3 (score 0), dilation 4 centimeters (score 2), no previous breech babies (score 0), would have a total score of five. A score of less than three would indicate the need for a cesarean section. A score of four to five indicates a careful review needs to be made and suggests one should proceed with caution. A score of five or more would indicate a reasonable chance for a successful vaginal delivery. Of course, some moderating factors exist. If a multipara has had two 9 pound babies vaginally and this baby is of similar size, she should do fine as long as the baby does not go postdates. I usually subtract one point for footling breeches, as they are somewhat more difficult to manage. In general, I have found this system to be very reliable for predicting outcome.

Breech Index Scoring System			
	0	1	2
Parity		Prime	Multip
Gestational Age	>39 wks.	37-38 wks.	36-37 wks.
Est. Fetal Weight	>8 lbs.	7-8 lbs.	5-7 lbs.
Dilation	2 cms	3 cms	>4 cms
Station	-3	-2	<-1
Previous Breech	0	1	>2

Breech Labor: What to Expect

The breech labor is in itself different from the vertex labor, and it deserves comment. In knowing what to expect, the midwife may free herself and her client from unnecessary concern and be more ready to recognize and assess abnormal progress, should it occur.

It is not unusual for the **waters to break prematurely**, especially in footling breeches. It is important to check for fetal heart tones immediately, in the event the cord is compromised or prolapsed.

It is common for the mother to go into labor anytime after **37 weeks' gestation**.

A fairly **long prodromal period** may be expected due to the lack of application of the presenting part to the cervix.

The mother usually experiences a **backache** of greater intensity than the abdominal pain, but less severe or persistent than with a posterior presentation.

Multiparous mothers with babies in the breech position may exhibit little or **no discomfort** in early labor and are often more than 4 centimeters dilated before they are aware of labor.

The mother may feel **"breathless"** during or after contractions due to pressure from the baby's head against the diaphragm.

Labor may **escalate abruptly** after the onset of active labor. This is often a surprise to the mother who thinks that this labor will be a "snap."

The mother often has an **early desire to push**, markedly more so with a footling breech.

There may be a **latent phase between complete dilation** and the expulsive stage of labor; the mother may even take a little nap when complete, which is to everyone's advantage.

(Continued on next page)

Tips & Tricks

Fluid Barrier
I put a cloth over the baby's face when just its head has been born. So often a gush of fluid—whether it is clear or stained, or blood—follows the body. Holding the cloth over the baby's face helps prevent intake of the fluids into the baby's lungs as the baby takes its first breath. Wiping the baby's mouth, then suctioning only if necessary, follows.

Shannon Brophy, America Online

Accentuate the Positive
Unless I hear fear or sounds that tell me a birthing woman is totally out of control, I tell clients who are embarrassed about moans and groans during birth that the pressure cooker would explode if not "allowed" to moan as it cooks. When I hear fear or out-of-control sounds, I encourage the woman to bring them into a controlled realm of constructive moaning.

One woman sat on the toilet during transition, and as a contraction intensified, her voice reflected the rise in intensity as she repeated over and over again, "Baby coming soon." Before that she had been quite fearful. Once she started to use a positive style, she progressed twice as fast.

Roberta Gehrke, MT

Be Patient
If a woman is infibulated, remember that the scar doesn't stretch. Let the second stage last as long as needed. Don't automatically reach for the scissors.

Mabel Dzata, OR

Back Labor
Use a rolling pin or paint roller over the woman's lower back for relief. You can also use counter pressure by pressing firmly with the palms of your hands on the area the mom directs you to. Don't worry about getting it right—she'll tell you! Remember that hot packs on the lower back can help relax the muscles.

Midwifery Today, Issue #46

Hands and Knees
When left on their own, most women deliver on hands and knees, where there is almost no risk of dangerous tears.

Michel Odent, London, UK

Tips & Tricks

Tricks for Prolonged Labor

For a long, prodromal labor, put a woman to sleep with a warm oil massage and one dropperful of valerian tincture. Chances are she will awaken two to three hours later with strong, effective contractions that will lead to birth.

Try warm water immersion; it relaxes a woman's body and helps her give in to her contractions. This simple, enjoyable technique will often speed up labor if the woman is five or more centimeters dilated. If she is less than five centimeters, help her get some rest.

Jill Cohen, OR

Sometimes prolonged labor calls for the "take charge routine." Move in close and do all you can to help the mother until she regains her inner strength. This technique is used for long labors where there are emotional lows, despair or a feeling of giving up.

Movement and position changes are essential tools in labor. When a woman is free to move around or lie down when she wants to, especially in long labors, it helps change the atmosphere and the diameter of the pelvis that the baby is moving through. It also helps the woman cope. Women know what to do in birth. We simply follow that through with them.

from The Birth Partner, by Penny Simkin

Visualization can open a cervix to 10 centimeters. Some women picture a flower opening.

Suggest to the birthing mother that she talk to her cervix and tell it to open. This is a good example of mind over matter.

Being present at a long labor is the most effective and soothing remedy I know for the birthing mother. A midwife's one-on-one care for however long it takes will help affirm her trust in you, herself and the process, and result in a good and safe birth.

Midwifery Today, Issue #46

Relaxing the Perineum

Support the birthing woman's legs completely in order to release tension. This relaxes the perineum.

Kathi Fox, CA

Multiparous mothers need lots of **reassurance** because breech descent feels very different from the vertex.

Meconium show is to be expected in second stage, particularly with "buttlings." Although this is normal, continue to assess heart tones continuously to rule out cord compromise.

Second stage contractions often do not last as long, nor are they as strong or frequent, as first stage contractions.

The presenting part is often **discolored**, and may appear **swollen**. This is no cause for alarm, as discoloration and swelling will disappear rapidly after birth.

It is normal for the baby to need a minute's rest before "**coming around.**" He has not had the scalp stimulation that occurs with the vertex delivery.

How the Attendant May Assist

Give the mother **lots of reassurance** during prodromal or latent labor.

Stay with her continuously, even in early labor, and take **heart tones regularly,** as the cord may become compromised at any time.

To help prevent cord prolapse in a footling breech, do not encourage the mother to walk or stand. Having her **sit in the "tailor" position** in a comfortable chair, with her back well-supported, will assist the baby's buttocks to move down (more into a squatting position) and will enhance application to the cervix, thus guarding against possible cord prolapse.

Very **warm baths** are always a welcome labor assistance. If she is uncomfortable, try placing a hot water bottle against the mother's lower back while she is in the tub.

Hands-and-knees position or knee-chest will help when the mother has an **uncontrollable urge** to push prematurely.

In **footling breech** presentations, try to keep the feet within the vagina as long as possible. If the mother can't stand it any more and they slip out, be sure to keep them covered and warm to prevent premature respiratory stimulation. Do not rush the birth! When the feet emerge, be sure to check for the cord.

Let mom **sleep** if she wants to. No harm will be done if the cervix has a chance to further efface. Remember that correct assessment of dilation is difficult in breeches, especially with footlings. I opt for an "hour of patience" to assure complete dilation. (Go for 12 centimeters!) As always, if you can feel the cervix, she is not complete. Remember: The predominant reason for breech delivery failures—stuck heads—is due to premature pushing or incorrect assessment of complete dilation.

Give oxygen generously as needed during second stage, especially when mother begins continuous pushing.

Keep mother **well hydrated**. It is not unusual for the breech mother to refuse food, as the continuous pressure of the baby's head in the upper abdomen may make her feel nauseous.

The midwife must be an expert at performing **newborn resuscitation**. She must have oxygen on hand and a pair of blunt/sharp scissors in the event of emergency episiotomy.

The Breech Delivery

1. Have the mother use a semi-reclining position, with legs, back and head well supported. I find the side of the bed works the best. It affords ample room in which to work and enables the midwife to easily bring the mother's buttocks to the edge of the bed to let gravity assist in the delivery of the baby's body. As much as possible, the delivery needs to occur by the spontaneous expulsive efforts of the mother. In general, a hands-off attitude on the part of the birth attendant yields the best results. Don't stretch or work the vagina; leave everything alone to allow for further dilation of the cervix. Don't encourage the mother to push, but also

(Continued on next page)

don't prevent the natural physiologic pushing that she will do at this time. She must reserve her energy for the continuous pushing that will soon be necessary.

2. Keep your hands off of the baby until you can "hang your hat on the butt," or until the baby is born to the navel. Once the presenting part emerges to this point, mother should push continuously, with or without contractions, until the baby is born completely. Never pull on the baby or try to free the legs until the body is born to the navel.

3. Once the navel has appeared pull down a loop of cord so that there will be no strain on the baby's navel. Gently touch the cord (do not pinch) to assess cord pulse. At this point, the baby must be born quickly. Stay calm! It is possible for the baby to suffocate if not born within 5 minutes. Please note: Time seems to stand still when we are under stress. Two minutes can seem like 20 minutes, so have an assistant keep track of the time.

4. Bring both legs down and out, one at a time. Remember to go with the bend of the knee. If the birth from the navel to armpit is not accomplished with the next contraction, gentle traction on the legs may be helpful. Don't be tempted to grasp the baby's body, as kidney damage may result. Be sure to keep the baby's back toward the mother's stomach. It is almost impossible to deliver a posterior breech (baby's back to mother's back) without damage. If you must assist the baby's rotation to anterior, do so by using both hands like splints, one on top, the other beneath, and gently turn both hands over, rotating the baby's body as you do so. Now bring the mother's buttocks over the edge of the bed, keeping her legs supported by assistants. The baby's body will drop down, easily exposing the nape of the neck and usually both arms will come down as well. Keeping one hand on the mother's perineum, grasp the baby's feet with the other hand and swing the body up and over onto the mother's abdomen. A towel or receiving blanket will help in holding onto the slippery body.

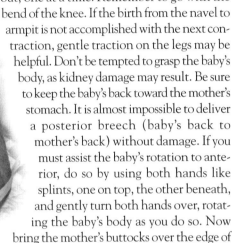

photo by Patti Ramos

5. Occasionally, the baby's arms will have been swept over its head. The baby will not be born if the arms and shoulders don't come down as the body emerges. If this happens, you must go inside the vagina and bring them down, one at a time. Do this by going up past the head, along the top of the shoulder, and hook a finger in the inside of the elbow and pull it down.

6. Have your assistant ready to apply supra-pubic pressure. As soon as the baby's mouth and nose appear, suction them. If necessary, pull the perineum down to establish an airway. Maintain perineal support and allow the rest of the head to be born slowly. If the baby is breathing, you have time to get the rest of the head out.

7. If the baby's head is not readily born, have an assistant apply supra-pubic pressure, cut an episiotomy and complete the delivery. (To avoid an episiotomy, I have often used the Ritgen Maneuver: I place my finger deeply into the mother's rectum and push the baby's head forward and out.) Never exert force by pulling on the baby's body while the head is still inside the mother. Doing so will cause irreparable damage to the baby's spinal cord, nervous system and breathing mechanism. When an airway has been established and the baby is breathing, he is in no danger, and further assistance may be summoned. Remember: damage is more often done by someone exerting too much force, than by the baby's being stuck. After the baby is born, have the mom give him a good rubbing, wrap him in a warm towel and keep a close eye on him. He hasn't had the massage that the

(Continued on next page)

Tips & Tricks

Nourishing Long Labors
It's important for the birthing woman to stay well hydrated and eat during a prolonged labor. Just a few bites and sips at a time can make a significant difference in how well the woman holds up. Miso soup with noodles makes an excellent long-labor snack, as does yogurt and fruit or honey. Popsicles made ahead of time from the juice of her choice can be appreciated, too. Recharge is a good beverage for long labors.

Midwifery Today, Issue # 46

Hands Off
Don't start perineal massage too soon. The mom may become swollen before you even see the baby's head. Tissue doesn't remain elastic. When elasticity is gone, she is bound to tear easily.

Tricks of the Trade Circle, NY '97

Telling the Truth
Some people are uncomfortable with the moaning and groaning women do while they give birth. One of my nurses ran into my room when I was making a lot of noise during transition and asked, "What's wrong?" My husband calmly said, "She's having a baby." Good perspective!

Alexandra Gruber-Malkin, Internet

Cooling Packs
If a woman is vaginally edematous or has enlarged hemorrhoids, try using cold compresses instead of warm compresses when she is crowning. I keep a bowl of ice water with a squirt of hibiscus in it and some washcloths handy. I use these to reduce swelling and cool down her "ring of fire." My women love it!

Christina Di Eno, FL

Low Tear Rate
At a Midwifery Today conference on waterbirth that was held in London, many practitioners presented very low tear rates with waterbirth. I asked an Austrian doctor why he thought that was so. He said the water provides the perfect amount of counterpressure.

Jan Tritten, OR

Tips & Tricks

Long Perineums
When discussing with another midwife the long perineum that always seems to tear, she suggested that the mom get into the hands-and-knees position. Last time I had such a mom, I tried it and the mom didn't tear. I think this position takes some of the stress off the perineum and positions the baby higher in the introitus.

Gail Hart (E-News)

Spontaneous Pushing
Telling someone not to push comes under my definition of coached pushing. Many of "my" moms—especially multips—push before full dilation and simply open up and give birth. If there is spontaneous bearing down, I'm inclined to leave it alone and just ask them how it feels. If it's really too soon, it hurts, and they're willing to back off. I usually don't even do a vaginal check (to evaluate for "complete dilation") unless it's not working. The most frequent reason for a vaginal check at that time is moms who think they aren't "allowed" to push until the magic 10 because of previous birth experience and/or training.

Kip Kozlowski (E-News)

A Minty Relief
Add one tablespoon peppermint extract or tincture to 4 ounces aloe vera gel; apply it to the birthing mother's perineum when she feels the burn of crowning. It is well absorbed by tissue and promotes tissue healing after birth. It also helps decrease swelling.

Julie Williams, CNM, MI

Rotating an OP Baby
To rotate an occipitoposterior baby, put the mother on her side in Trendelenburg's position (supine on a table that is tilted head downward 45 degrees or less). The first time I tried it, the baby rotated and delivered quickly. It probably gets the baby's head "unstuck" from the birth canal and helps it rotate easier. Most others can tolerate this position better than knee-chest, and it seems to work better. We put a large wedge under the mattress of the bed. A bean bag could also work.

Margie Riley

---

vertex baby has had during labor, so he usually needs almost a full minute to get going. I often score the baby's Apgar at intervals of one, two and five minutes. You may find that if the baby has been within his mother with his feet up over his head, he will most likely lie the same way now, causing him to look like a little frog! Sometimes, baby boys present scrotum first, causing it to become very swollen and purple. Reassure the dad that the damage is temporary.

I do not advocate the squatting position for breech delivery for four very important reasons:

- I do not want the birth to happen quickly. Head decompression can lead to subdural hemorrhage.
- Squatting may cause the baby's arms to be swept up over its head, f further complicating the delivery and possibly causing Erb's paralysis during the extraction of the arms.
- The baby's body hangs straight down, causing an almost military emergence of the head, which exerts undue pressure on the base of the baby's neck and increases the risk of spinal cord damage.
- The mother's perineum will tear at a much higher rate.

It was my desire to illustrate in this article what may be expected in a normal breech labor, the ideal management of breech labor and delivery, how to assess risk factors in determining feasibility of attempted delivery, and recognition of true complications. We must prepare in advance for a safe delivery, both physically and psychologically.

All in all, I do not consider the breech delivery to be either steeped in mystery or terrifying. It is a very special event which deserves both respectful and intelligent consideration so that a happy outcome may be achieved for both mother and baby.

Editor's Note: *As Valerie states in her article, breech births are special events. However, they do take a great deal of study, knowledge and hands-on experience to ensure safe and happy outcomes for families. Please do not feel that this article will qualify you to attempt a breech delivery without further study.*

Increased Comfort in the Squatting Position.

A variety of stools are available in many shapes, as convertible birth chairs, even rockers.

"One of the principal protagonists of non-interventionist childbirth is the South American obstetric physiologist Caldeyro-Barcia, who has demonstrated scientifically the physiological benefit of natural labour and birth.

"He also shows that delivery on a birth chair, which prevents supine hypotensive syndrome and compression in the diaphragm, increases placental perfusion and fetal oxygenation and that in this position blood gases remain satisfactory even if second stage lasts 120 minutes, providing organised breath holding and pushing session are avoided. He found that on the whole with the mother sitting or squatting, the delivery phase is shortened by both gravity and the increase in pelvic capacity."

From Midwives in History and Society, *by J. Fowler and J. Bramall*

"In the Western World, the stool or chair remained indispensably part of the equipment of most midwives up to the middle of the 18th century. Each wealthy household had its own stool, while among the poor, a stool was transported from house to house. The birth stools of royalty were carved and ornamented with jewels.... Even today, a birth chair is still used by some Egyptian women."

From New Life, *by Janet Balaskas*

Immediate Postpartum

How Long Is Too long?

by Gail Hart, Midwife

AFTER A VERY normal labor (four-hour first stage, 15-minute transition, one-minute second stage), my client had a prolonged third stage. Her uterus was firm, central, globular, at the navel. It was not rising or filling with blood or clots. She had no sign of placental separation: no change in shape of uterus, no bleeding or lengthening of the cord. She had no contractions and was enjoying and nursing her baby.

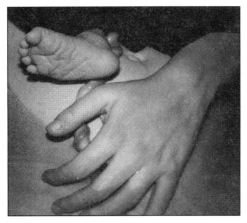
photo by Patti Ramos

After 30 minutes, I advised her to change positions and also empty her bladder, if she felt able. She did this willingly, but in spite of increased activity, a vertical position and an empty bladder, she still had no contractions or signs of placental separation.

At 50 minutes postpartum, I told my client she was going beyond the usual time guidelines for third-stage labor. Further, I told her protocols drafted by my state organization advised transport to a hospital for delivery of the placenta. (My state guidelines later called for mandatory transport in this situation.)

We discussed the use of herbs and Pitocin. She agreed to try the herbs angelica, shepherd's purse, and blue and black cohosh, but flatly refused an injection of Pitocin. She also refused transport. She told me her placentas "always take a long time to come" and said the only time she had ever had difficulty was when someone tried to hurry the delivery.

She took the herbs with no visible effect. We continued to monitor her uterus for signs of placental separation or hidden bleeding. Her pulse and blood pressure were stable, and she was getting annoyed with me for being overly concerned about the situation.

At one hour and 40 minutes postpartum, she took a warm shower and said she was having a contraction. She squatted on the shower floor and I noticed a small amount of blood (perhaps 50 cc). I asked her to return to the bed. Upon examination, I found her uterus was narrow, and had risen in her right side, and the umbilical cord had lengthened. When she had her next contraction five minutes later, she pushed and delivered her placenta. The total blood loss in this labor was well under three-quarters of a cup.

On three other occasions, I have seen this same pattern of delayed contractions leading to a prolonged third stage. I know that most doctors, and even some midwives, would feel more comfortable intervening, perhaps by using drugs to start contractions, or by attempting to separate and deliver the placenta manually. But when the placenta is clearly not separated, the uterus has no contraction pattern, and the mother is not bleeding, I believe the risks of interference are much greater than the risks of waiting for the uterus to work on its own. I would rather wait for a slow placenta than cause a partial separation and hemorrhage.

Wise birth practitioners know timetables are arbitrary. A two-hour second stage is average. But as we as all know, each woman is unique and each birth is a unique situation. While two hours may be adequate for some women, other women need much more time for second stage. When we intervene unnecessarily, we may cause a far greater problem than the one we're attempting to fix.

The bottom line, as always, is that the condition of the mother and baby is the only factor that really matters when making the judgment "how long is too long?"

Tips & Tricks
Facilitating Third Stage

I often "talk to" the placenta, thanking "Madame Placenta" for its wonderful function, "and now, would you please come out?" I think this calms me down (if it's a long third stage) and it calms the family and adds a little humor to an otherwise tense situation.

Annette Manant, CNM (E-news)

Get the mother in the hands-and-knees position while in the tub or shower. Run the shower massage up and down her back, have her do pelvic rocks, then get her to sit on the toilet.

Laura, Maui, HI

Have the mother put her thumb in her mouth and blow hard.

Gladys Milton, FL

Use words of love. Mother and midwife look at each other like lovers.

Naolí Vinaver, Mexico

The Nepalese put a bus token in a mixture of sugar and water; drinking the mixture helps "drive the placenta out."

Sara Wu, OR

Lava Lamp

I had a client who had had a retained placenta with her first baby. During one of our prenatal visits, she mentioned her friend had a lava lamp, and she was finding it to be a great visualization aid for plopping out her placenta. After she birthed her daughter I reminded her she wasn't finished with her work. She relaxed and said, "Lava Lamp," and out came the placenta.

Janneli, AOL

Ice Packs

In Russia they used ice packs on the uterus to contract it and stop postpartum hemorrhage. It worked!

Jill Cohen, OR

Hemorrhoid Prevention and Treatment

by Roberta Gehrke, CNM

MOST OF MY BOOKS say that hemorrhoids are started by constipation during pregnancy and are aggravated by the pushing stage. So prevention could be the key—a gentle pushing stage in positions that keep the woman off her back and keep her bottom from being compressed between the bed and the baby's head. When a woman is allowed to labor her way—according to need and in a variety of positions—does she have a better chance of preventing hemorrhoids?

I like to have women deliver on their left side if possible. I prepare a soft paper towel with the kind of aloe gel that is used for sunburn. With the toweling over the heel of my left hand, I apply gentle counterpressure as the mom pushes—it will keep even the largest hemorrhoids from swelling too much as the baby descends.

Immediately after the birth, any external bulges that will retract should be pushed into the rectum beyond the sphincter muscle. Applying the same kind of aloe gel during this procedure numbs the area and makes the job easier. Then bring the mother's legs down and apply a previously prepared icepack made from a condom half filled with water and wrapped in another paper towel and frozen. The woman should retract the hemorrhoids each time she uses the bathroom. Wiping with a baby wipe with aloe eliminates the itching and burning. If the hemorrhoids have been left out, the sphincter acts like a rubber band around them and they become even more swollen.

If clots have formed, the homeopathic remedy, Bothrops 30x, works miracles. It is taken a pellet or two at a time when pain occurs. At first the pain may occur every 10 minutes, but the intervals extend as the clot disintegrates. If a doctor insists on removing the clot (the only method doctors know), make sure he goes up into the varicosed vessel and removes any small clots. Otherwise the small ones up inside will continue to descend, and like snowballs, they will become bigger if not removed.

If a woman's hemorrhoids swell, ask her to wash and grate a potato, making sure there is some peel included. Scoop it into a 1-1/2 inch pile, one-quarter inch thick in the middle of a paper towel. Twist the towel to make a small pouch. Tell the woman to place the single side of the towel next to the rectum and slip on her panties. It will take just a matter of minutes for the woman to feel much more comfortable and a couple of days for the swelling to diminish.

Controlled Cord Traction

by Roberta Gehrke, CNM

IF YOU HAVE EVER seen a uterine prolapse with all its ramifications and hemorrhage, you will not doubt the value of guarding the uterus. To this day I remember how placenta delivery techniques were taught to me when I was studying basic midwifery in London 20 years ago. I recall the demonstration with a smile every time my hand goes to a uterus after the birth of a babe and before the placenta comes out.

The Sister asked one of my classmates to stand up and put her arms out; she threw a sheet over her and said, "This is the uterus, tubes and ovaries." She then jabbed the student moderately firmly in the sides, making her jump and quickly bring down her arms. Sister then said, "When you are getting impatient waiting for the placenta to let loose, the first rule is to never fiddle with the fundus! It makes the uterus jumpy, and it clamps down, keeping the placenta trapped for longer than it needs to be. It can lead to hidden hemorrhage between the placenta and uterine wall."

Gently feel the fundus and sides of the uterus for the contour to change shape from round and low to narrow and higher in the abdomen. Then bring your hand to the pubic bone, placing the little finger side of your hand between the top edge of the pubic bone and the lower edge of the uterus as you do gentle cord traction. I prefer to do the traction with my fingers instead of forceps. The cord is slippery and using my fingers keeps me from becoming too vigorous in my pull. It also helps me feel for the first hint of tearing of the cord from the placenta.

Uterine prolapse is rare, thank goodness, possibly because our training has indoctrinated us to guard the woman's body during the process of delivery. If nothing else, the fact that the uterus is capable of prolapsing is a constant reminder to be gentle. It also reminds us to keep a hand in place to hold the uterus above the pelvis so that it will not bleed as heavily as it would if allowed to descend into the wide-open spaces now available there. The other hand goes to the fundus as soon as the placenta/membranes are all out to make sure the uterus is firm: "like your knee, not like your thigh," as I tell the mother.

Postpartum Bleeding

by Gert Welsh, CNM

AFTER MANY YEARS as a midwife I realized that I feared third stage labor. Grand multiparas would often deliver on contractions that were anywhere from five to 10 minutes apart. Immediately after the delivery, contractions were still that far apart but were enough to partially separate the placenta, and the bleeding would start. It was very hard to be cool and relaxed with all that blood pouring out and a baby who wasn't quite ready to nurse.

Years ago we didn't do much nipple stimulation to start contractions, so I turned to oxytocics for help. Since postpartum bleeding was a frequent problem and we were assisting women in a small rural clinic 20 miles from the nearest hospital, we started IVs on most women so we'd have an open vein "when the bleeding started."

As time progressed, I challenged myself to get over my "placenta wars." I have become very alert to indications that the placenta may continue its assaults on my skills. After all, it is not a "beast" but a wonderful, nourishing organ that helps moms grow lovely babies.

I ask the placenta to tell me where it is located. Do I hear the souffle moving upward during my prenatal checks? Did I get an ultrasound? Where is the placenta located? Are there any fibroids? Is there a septum in the uterus? Any of these conditions can cause excessive bleeding because they interfere with the normal constriction of uterine blood vessels in the placental bed.

Often when these things are present, I need to be alert at the time of the birth to be certain that the placenta separates in a timely fashion. Once the placenta is out, if bleeding or oozing is heavy and there are no lacerations or other causes of bleeding, the first thing I do is elevate the uterus as high in the abdomen as I can. Second, I do bimanual compression through the abdominal wall by elevating the uterus and then compressing it between my two hands. (A generous amount of verbal anesthesia is required here.) If this is not possible, I use a vaginal hand to elevate the uterus and then compress it between the abdominal and vaginal hands.

At the same time either nipple stimulation by the baby licking or sucking, or nipple rolling is done. If there isn't an IV in place and bleeding is brisk, an IV is started. Pitocin is added for frequent contractions and/or Methergine is administered intramuscularly for longer, stronger contractions. One can also give Pitocin intravenously, though we were taught in the old school to barrage it in by injecting a small amount, withdrawing some blood to mix with the Pitocin and dilute it, and then injecting a bit more until 10 units are injected.

Another technique I frequently use for heavy oozing in a previously well-contracted uterus is to gently insert two fingers into the cervix and ream any clots from it. I have noticed that when the cervix is held open by clots, the lower uterine segment fills with clots and continues to ooze. Clots can also build up behind the cervix in the vaginal vault. In retrospect, I note that low-lying placentas frequently leave very wet placental beds that ooze, and the cervix will contain clots. Elevating and holding the uterus constricts the uterine arteries and decreases bleeding. It also stretches the round ligaments and causes increased fundal contractions. This helps contract the vertical muscular fibers of the lower uterine segment and will decrease the wetness factor.

Another way to keep the uterus elevated that works very well is the placement of a 1-pound weight above the symphysis and below the uterus. Through the years, workshop and class participants have told me they have successfully used 1-pound traction weights or sandbags. Another idea is to use frozen bottles—empty rectangular-shaped rubbing alcohol bottles that have been filled with water and stored in the freezer.

When all is said and done, the best defense is a great offense. My favorite offense is to keep good contraction patterns going in labor by feeding, hydrating and resting the laboring mom. I also ask her to be active by walking, standing, sitting on a birthing ball or in a rocking chair, slow dancing with her partner or other support person, swaying side to side as she leans over the bed supported on her elbows, or using water therapy in the shower or tub. It's a shame that a woman who has just given birth and is enjoying her baby has to be distressed by vigorous uterine massage. While I try not to do that, I have a rule that says, "Nobody bleeds too much."

Tips & Tricks

C-section Scar
Keep in mind that with a woman who has had a previous cesarean, part of the placenta may be stuck in a pocket at the site of the scar.
Naolí Vinaver, Mexico

Focus on Baby
If you have to do a manual removal of the placenta, tell the mother to look at the baby while it is being done. Concentrating on the baby will help her to cope with pain or discomfort.
Abby Odam, CA

Time Warp
When a baby is just born, remember that 60 to 90 seconds for the baby to start is pretty normal. Time seems to stand still; just keep cool.
Debbie Diáz Ortiz, Puerto Rico

Warm Receiving Blankets
A buffet plate warmer is like a long heating pad on which a plate is placed and the pad is folded over it, another plate is placed, the pad is folded, and so on. When the laboring mom starts to push, we place receiving blankets in the folds instead. By the time the baby is born the blankets are toasty warm.
Cher Simnitt, CA

Postpartum Hemorrhage
If the woman has a history of postpartum hemorrhage, I will often offer her shepherd's purse tincture prophylactically, two droppersful under the tongue after the placenta delivers. Have her hold it under the tongue as long as she can stand it, then follow with a little bit of water to drink.
Annette Manant, CNM (E-News)

Can We Really Use Super Glue Instead of Suture?

by Anne Frye, CPM

FOR SEVERAL YEARS, there has been increasing interest in the midwifery community regarding the use of commonly available "Super Glue" types of adhesives for wound closure. Midwives who have done a little research have found the cyanoacrylate glue sold over the counter apparently identical in composition to medical cyanoacrylate glues. The over-the-counter brand is also rumored to be the same as the tissue adhesive used extensively during the Vietnam War. Some midwives have even used Super Glue (Krazy Glue) successfully in lieu of suture to close the perineum.

In revising my book *Healing Passage: A Midwife's Guide to the Care and Repair of the Tissues Involved in Birth*, I felt it was important to address this issue. This article offers an expanded version of the information you will find in the new fifth edition.

History and Development

In 1959, a variety of cyanoacrylate adhesives were developed. Some of these are now used for surgical purposes in Canada and Europe. These glues polymerize on contact with basic substances, such as water or blood, to form a strong bond. The first glue developed was methyl cyanoacrylate, which was studied extensively for its potential medical applications and was rejected due to its potential tissue toxicity, such as inflammation or local foreign body reactions. Methyl alcohol has a short molecular chain, which contributes to these complications.

Further research revealed that by changing the type of alcohol in the compound to one with a longer molecular chain, the tissue toxicity was greatly reduced. All the medical grade tissue adhesives currently available for human use contain butyl-esters, which are costlier to produce.

In 1964, the Tennessee Eastman lab submitted to the FDA its first application for new drug approval. The military learned of this new glue and became extremely interested in its potential for use in field hospitals. MASH units in Vietnam were overloaded. Many soldiers were dying from chest and abdominal wounds despite the best efforts of medics. In 1966, a special surgical team was flown to Vietnam, where it was trained and equipped to use cyanoacrylate adhesive. A quick spray over the wounds stopped bleeding and bought the patient time until conventional surgery could be performed. The possibilities were immediately seized by the medical communities of Europe and the Far East. Meanwhile, the FDA changed standards and kept requesting additional data until Eastman was reluctantly forced to withdraw its application.

Histoacryl Blue (n-butyl cyanoacrylate) has been used extensively in Europe since the 1970s for a variety of surgical applications, including middle ear surgery, bone and cartilage grafts, repair of cerebrospinal fluid leaks, and skin closure. It has been available in Canada through Davis & Geck Canada, with no adverse effects reported to date. Further, laboratory studies have been done which concluded that it has no carcinogenic potential. Tissue toxicity has been noted only when the adhesive is introduced deep in highly vascular areas (the perineum qualifies as such an area). While I always take claims of harmlessness with a grain of salt, these adhesives appear to be basically safe if used as directed.

An interesting note on this point is that Hulda Clark, a naturopath who has done extensive research on the correlation of toxic substances in the body with various disease conditions, has found that propyl alcohol and wood alcohol are related to the development of cancer and diabetes, respectively. Therefore, the use of an alcohol-based product may well be questionable.

Current Use

Although not labeled as such, over-the-counter Super Glue products contain methyl alcohol because it is inexpensive to produce. Cyanoacrylates cure by a chemical reaction called polymerization, which produces heat. Methyl alcohol has a pronounced heating action when it touches tissue and may even produce burns if the glue comes in contact with a large enough area of tissue. Rapid curing may also lead to tissue necrosis. Midwives have not noted such reactions because minimal amounts are being used for perineal repair. Nevertheless, due to the toxic potential, over-the-counter products are inappropriate for use in wound closure.

Medical grade products currently available contain either butyl, isobutyl or octyl esters. They are bacteriostatic and painless to apply when used as directed. Also, they produce minimal thermal reaction when applied to dry skin and break down harmlessly in tissue. They are essentially inert once dry. Butyl products are rigid when dry, but provide a strong bond. Available octyl products are more flexible when dry, but produce a weaker bond.

When used for repair, the wound to be closed is ideally fresh, clean, fairly shallow, with straight edges that lie together on their own. The glue is applied to bridge over the closed edges; it should not be used within the wound (on raw surfaces), where it will impair epithelization. The only currently FDA-approved

(Continued on next page)

(Continued from previous page)
adhesives suitable for use as suture alternatives are veterinary products: n-butyl-cyanoacrylate tissue adhesives Vetbond (3M) and Nexaband liquid and octyl-based Nexaband S/C (intended for topical skin closure when deep sutures have been placed).

Histoacryl Blue (butyl-based) (Davis & Geck) and Tissu-Glu (isobutyl-based) (Medi-West Pharmaceuticals) are sold in Canada for human use. DMSO (dimethyl sulfoxide) or acetone serves as removers.

How to Use Tissue Adhesive

Although not specifically recommended for perineal repair, tissue adhesive has been used successfully by some midwives. However, Histoacryl Blue was used in place of interrupted or subcuticular stitches in a small study of the closure of the superficial layer in mediolateral clitorotomy (episiotomy). In this study, the yoni (vaginal) mucosa and subcutaneous layers were closed with conventional suture techniques. It might be a good alternative to offer when women refuse conventional sutures.

Tissue adhesive works best when the wound is moderately shallow. Midwives report that extremely shallow wounds tend to pull apart as healing occurs and usually require no closure of any kind. The wound should also have no pockets to collect lochia and should not require other sutures. However, as this study demonstrates, it can also be used instead of subcuticular sutures after placing basting stitches.

Tissue glue is applied only to outside surfaces to bridge over edges; do not apply it directly to raw surfaces.

The wound edges should be straight and lie together naturally. Insert a tampon, then clean and dry the skin thoroughly. Have your assistant stabilize the wound edges from top to bottom (be sure the edges are matched correctly).

Insert your finger between the edges and pull it out to bring the edges forward slightly. This is to ensure that the wound edges are not rolled inward toward each other, but meet perfectly. It could also be accomplished with a tissue forceps. Hold gauze against the area immediately below the apex to catch any drips as you apply the glue. Apply tiny dots of glue sparingly at intervals where the wound edges meet. Or, apply a bead of tiny droplets to bridge the edges. (Thick applications do not enhance bonding and tend to crack and loosen prematurely.) Products dyed blue are easier to see. (If using Histoacryl Blue, attach a 27-gram syringe needle to the ampule hub to help control application. After use, the needle should be discarded and replaced with a new needle that does not have glue within its lumen.) Be careful to apply the glue only where it is needed; glue removers should not be used in the genital area. As long as no part of the tube tip or the attached needle contacts the tissue or bodily fluids, the tube can be reused.

Use a hair dryer or fan the area dry; it will take about 30 seconds. The adhesive will stiffen when dry. Women should observe the same precautions as those who have refused sutures entirely. Bathing is not contraindicated, but prolonged soaking should be avoided. Expect the adhesive to flake off in three to seven days. Allergic reactions are very rare, but may include inflammation and swelling.

References
Adoni, A., and Anteby, E. (1991, May). The use of histoacryl for episiotomy repair. *British Journal of Obstetrics and Gynecology.* 98: 476-8.
Clark, Hulda. (1995). *The Cure for All Diseases.* San Diego: ProMotion Publishing.
Heimstetter, G. (1995). Personal communication, Permabond International, Bridgewater, N.J.
Jueneman, F. (1981, Aug.). Stick it to um. *Industrial Research & Dev.:* p. 19.
Quinn, J., and Kissack, J. (1994). Tissue adhesives for laceration repair during sporting events. *Clinical Journal of Sports Medicine* 4(4): 245

Sources for tissue adhesives
Animal Care Products, 3M Health Care, 3M Center Building 225 1N 07, St. Paul, MN 55144-1000, (612) 733-8477. 3M produces Vetbond Tissue Adhesive.
Veterinary Products Laboratory, (800)548-2828, distributes Nexaband products that are manufactured by Tri-Point in Raleigh, NC, (919) 790-1041. These products are restricted items sold and approved for veterinary use only.
Davis & Geck Canada, (905) 4703647, distributes Histoacryl Blue, which is manufactured in Germany by B. Braun.
Medi-West Pharmaceuticals markets Tissu-Glu.

Tips & Tricks
Tears/Healing
If a midwife and mom decide to leave a second- or third-degree tear to heal on its own, they should remember it will heal from the bottom up and the inside out. It looks scary for a couple of days, but it will heal and look normal.
Tricks of the Trade Circle, Ann Arbor '96

A postpartum ginger sitz bath is wonderfully relaxing and pleasant and helps ease pain or discomfort. Ginger also stimulates blood flow to the perineum to hasten healing.
Elizabeth Chace, MA

Have the mother put one-half teaspoon of blue chamomile oil in her bath to help heal sutures.
Barbara Kircher, Buttlar, Germany

To Sew or Not?
I am in strong favor of not suturing first- and second-degree tears! In Scotland where I trained, many midwives were adopting the practice of not suturing first- and second-degree tears that approximate nicely and aren't actively bleeding. If it is questionable, leave a pad on, legs together for a while, then take a look. It is often remarkable how quickly a tear goes from looking pretty bad to "leavable."

When you decide to leave it (and, of course, discuss the options with the mother—I bet she'll opt for no suturing), give her some advice (e.g., arnica for swelling and bruising, frequent cleansing, lavender/tea tree baths). Explain that it will probably take a full six weeks to come together completely, then don't examine *every* day as long she is comfortable, but keep an eye on it (or teach your client how to).

My baby was born at home after one of those marathon labors. I had a second-degree tear, and it would have been a terrible thing to endure getting sutured after all that! Instead, my midwife left it, I got to enjoy my first minutes with my daughter, and I healed beautifully!
Amy Darling (E-News)

The Vitamin K Question

If It Ain't Broke ...

I read with interest Jennifer Enoch's well-researched, thought-provoking article (*Midwifery Today*, Issue No. 40) urging newborn vitamin K prophylaxis. Yet, I concur with Nancy Wainer's and Cathy O'Bryant's comments ("Networking," *Midwifery Today*, Issue No. 41) when they remind us that a vast majority of babies are born complete, whole and ready to go. They need no special additives, just liberal doses of colostrum, breast milk and love.

In my 16 years of practice, I have resisted the pressure to tinker with the intricate integrity of newborn physiology. Only very rarely—such as if a baby has had serious birth trauma, was born quite early, or has a manifest defect or injury—do I even consider administering anything. If, under the circumstances, administering vitamin K seems prudent, then I use an oral form. Should reasons for concern arise later in a previously normal newborn (oozing cord, significant bruising, unusual petechiae, bloody stool and so forth), treatment may clearly be indicated.

Yet, it is my opinion that well-nourished, informed, attentive, drug-free mothers can appropriately, in good conscience, decline routine newborn vitamin K injections. In my practice, I have observed only minimally diminished clotting in one infant born without a pituitary gland and a fetal alcohol syndrome (FAS) 35-1/2 week preemie (both were treated empirically with vitamin K given orally in the first 24 hours with apparent success). My clients and I are, nevertheless, vigilant for any indication that normalcy has been compromised, so we can ameliorate the problem. In the meantime, though, my approach is, "If it ain't broke, don't fix it."

Judy Edmunds, Bellingham, WA

Forms of Vitamin K

I am concerned about the article on vitamin K. There are two forms of natural vitamin K: phytonadione or phylloqinone (K1) from plants, and menaquinone (K2), manufactured by bacteria in the large intestine. Konakion, made by Roche Laboratories, is not "phylloqinone, a natural form of vitamin K." According to Roche's insert, Konakion is "phytomenadione, a synthetic preparation of vitamin Kl." Information in their Netherlands oral preparation also acknowledges that the active ingredient is fyto (phyto) menadion, "a synthetically made vitamin K."

The Merck Index, 11th edition, gives the following description: "menadione, a synthetic napthoquinone derivative having the physiologic properties of vitamin K."

Naptho-quinones are from the same family of petrochemicals as phthalates (xeno-oestrogens) recently implicated in nine brands of U.K. infant formulae linked to declining sperm levels and testicular abnormalities.

A 1992 position statement from Roche Australia in regard to using Konakion injections as an oral route administration said, "We have no clinical studies to support the use of Kanakion ampoules solution being given orally....Vitamin K in injection is preserved with phenol which has been reported to be an irritant on neonatal mucosa....For the above reasons we would not recommend the administration of Konakion ampoule solution orally to neonates."

Joan Donley, Auckland, Australia

Risk and Prevention

I am presently developing a research, project on vitamin K prophylaxis for my master's thesis. I would like to add some further information and clarification for the benefit of midwives and families.

Breast milk and vitamin K: I would argue very strongly that breast milk does contain sufficient vitamin K (VK) for most newborns. Human milk contains 2-15 ug/ml of VK. Breast hind milk contains larger amounts of VK, but infant intake is reduced in the first days of life. Two studies have shown that a breast-fed infant may receive less than 0.5 ug/ml of VK in the first three days of life, while an artificially fed infant will take in up to 50 ug/ml. The majority of exclusively breast-fed infants reaches adult levels of VK by day four or five and does not develop late hemorrhagic disease of the newborn (LHDN). Therefore, the daily requirement of VK is probably very small, or the VK in breastmilk is better absorbed.

Maternal vitamin K supplements: One study linked socioeconomic deprivation to an increased risk of LHDN. Another study found data that suggested a dietary link: in Eastern Japan infants have a lower incidence of LHDN. Women in these areas eat more fermented soybeans (high in VK) than those from Western Japan, where there is a higher incidence of LHDN. However, in another study, analysis of the VK content in breast milk of mothers of affected and non-affected infants found no direct association with late LHDN and low VK levels in breast milk.

Risk factors for LHDN: When the infants with idiopathic LHDN are assessed, they often are diagnosed with liver disorders that reduce the production of bile salts. These liver disorders are mild and asymptomatic and usually resolve without incident, except in cases where the infants have not received M4 VK prophylaxis. Secondary LHDN is most commonly associated with diseases that affect the concentration of bile salts in the small intestine, such as cystic fibrosis, alpha-1 antitrypsin deficiency, and bile duct atresia. Studies of VK absorption after oral VK prophylaxis have highlighted the large variation in absorption between infants, pointing to individual differences in

VK absorption via the intestines.

Informed choice and LHDN: Midwives are responsible for providing women and their families with unbiased information in a non-authoritative manner so that they may make informed choices. It is essential that women and families make an informed choice regarding VK prophylaxis. When clients decline VK or choose the oral route, I emphasize the need for parents to watch for warning bleeds or bruising, as well as signs of LHDN. Most case studies refer to a warning bleed prior to the major episode, including bruising, nosebleeds, umbilical oozing or blood in the stool. In a recent study, seven out of 14 infants went on to have major intracranial hemorrhage (ICH) within one to 14 days following the warning bleed. Infants with LHDN usually present with shock, pallor, high-pitched crying, poor appetite, poor sucking, limp or floppy bodies, and a decrease in level of consciousness.

We have no way of telling which infant is at risk. There are two good choices for effective prophylaxis of LHDN. The first is an Rd injection of VK at birth, the second is oral VK at birth followed by weekly doses until three months or when exclusive breast-feeding is stopped.

Freda Seddon, RM, Ontario, Canada

Symptoms of HDN

- Bleeding from the umbilicus, nose, mouth, ears, urinary tract or rectum
- Any bruise that is not related to known trauma
- Petechiae (pinpoint bruises)
- Black, tarry stool (after the meconium) or black vomit, which may contain blood acted on by digestive enzymes and resulting from bleeding in the gastrointestinal tract
- Bleeding longer than six minutes from a blood sampling site despite application of pressure on the wound
- Symptoms of intracranial bleeding include: paleness, a glassy-eyed look, irritability or high-pitched crying, loss of appetite, vomiting, fever, prolonged jaundice.

Jennifer Enoch

Tips & Tricks

Tea Tree Oil for Wound
I am an aspiring midwifery student in Germany. The midwives and doctors here use tea tree oil on the suture wound. A few days after a woman has had an episiotomy or has torn, she is given a syringe with the needle still attached, filled with tea tree oil. She is then shown how to use a mirror to see her wound and to drop a few drops of this wonderfully cool oil directly on it. If she is not comfortable doing this, the postpartum midwife will apply the oil. Putting the oil in the syringe with needle allows accurate application. This is standard practice here, and from personal experience, I can attest that it really works well.

Kiersten Figurski (E-News)

Hemorrhoid Rx
To treat hemorrhoids: Grate one medium potato; mix well with 2-3 teaspoons slippery elm powder. Form into small patty and place on disturbed area for 10 to 15 minutes, one to three times a day. This remedy may be used on sore or cracked nipples as well.

Mary Bove, ND(E-News)

Incontinence
In many cases of mild to severe incontinence, and in several prolapse situations, I have found the rebounder to provide miraculous results. The uterus cannot prolapse if the pelvic floor is strong.

A rebounder is a small trampoline. Empty the bladder first, put on a pad (you will probably leak!), and begin gentle bounces. As you work up to more vigorous exercise, you will find the pelvic floor much strengthened and surgical repair unlikely to be necessary.

D. Parkin, R.M. (E-News)

Postpartum Depression
Few families readily perceive the full extent of a woman's vulnerability once labor has ceased. Many times, the intense focus and concentration that friends and family members direct toward the mother are abruptly withdrawn and transferred to the infant or elsewhere. Some women who are strongly dependent on this psychological/emotional support sense the loss acutely. This may contribute to postpartum depression.

Judy Edmunds in "The Grand Finale to Birth," Midwifery Today Issue No. 34

We've had a lot of success in our practice using breastfeeding itself as an antidepressant, with supporting herbs and very good nutrition to help manage overwhelm/fatigue/blues. We have used sedating teas: catnip, skullcap, licorice. We have used mood and hormone stabilizers in tincture form as needed: motherwort, dong quai, lemon balm. We have used Bach Flower Remedies as needed: olive and Rescue Remedy. Many mothers who previously used psych meds are skilled at determining when the herbs are not enough for them.

S. Condon, CNM, NY (E-News)

Patience!
Angelica tincture (also called dong quai) can be used after a birth to help release the placenta. Also make sure the vitamin E intake the last month before birth is no more than 400 IU daily. But patience is most important when waiting on the placenta. There will be a tendency to hurry the placenta out and that can definitely lead to hemorrhaging. Some placentas are much slower to detach than others, and pulling them off too soon is what actually causes the hemorrhaging.

Waiting patiently is actually the best treatment for accreta as long as blood loss is not excessive. But her care provider must be well aware of her previous history and have emergency plans in place.

J. Jones, CPM

Tips & Tricks

Suctioning, Or Not

I do not suction my babies routinely; I feel this procedure is a man-made thing. When I deliver my babies, I turn them over onto their stomachs with their heads down and brush up their backs and they will spit up what they need to. With suctioning of any kind, mucous is forced down the throat, as well as meconium. Unless you plan to intubate and suction with a vacuum tube, like in the hospital, the only meconium you will be suctioning will be down the esophagus. This is traumatic to the baby and throws him into the vagal response, which increases his respiration and heart rate at a critical time when he should be stabilizing.

I find that most of the meconium which babies will spit up is in a large mucous plug, tinged with the meconium, within the first six to eight hours after birth. If baby's respiration is slightly elevated from normal, a small amount of sterile water can be given to him, and he will soon spit up a large mucous plug and be just fine. If you are concerned that baby may have aspirated meconium, about the only thing you can do is watch for signs of infection if you do not plan to intubate and suction.

Cathy O'Bryant, (E-News)

Delay Cord Clamping

Something unheard of in hospital births: Not clamping or tying the cord at all and severing it only when it has completely stopped pulsating decreases the incidence of umbilical hernia (which I have seen in hospital clients' babies even with delayed clamping).

Connie Banack, (E-News)

A Relaxing Bath With Baby

Co-bathing is a good technique to use with babies who have had their natural instincts interfered with due to traumatic birth, vigorous suctioning, labor drugs, etc. The mother and baby have a nice, warm bath together with the baby positioned on the mother's tummy and an assistant gently pouring water over the baby to keep her warm. Many babies will actually "crawl" up the mother's body and self-attach to the breast, something that babies from non-traumatic, unmedicated births will do if allowed to soon after delivery. If self-attachment doesn't occur, then at least the mother and baby have had a lovely relaxing bath together.

Denise, Brisbane, Australia

Comfort First

I have my moms use undergarments designed for incontinence during the first three days after birth–they are more comfortable.

Carrie Abbott, UT

Retained Placenta

Use these homeopathic remedies:

Sabina 30c—This is useful for haemorrhage with retained placenta. It will promote expulsion. There may be watery blood with dark clots. The patient typically feels chilly, with cold hands and feet. Give every 10 minutes for four doses.

Secale 30c—Patient is relaxed and contractions have no expulsive action. Hourglass contractions. Haemorrhage with continual oozing of thin, dark-coloured blood. The patient is typically hot, wants fresh air and doesn't want to be covered. Give one dose every 10 to 20 minutes depending on situation.

Sepia 30c—For situations where there is back pain which is better for hard pressure in the small of the back. The Sepia patient has a tendency to prolapse and often has a history of severe "dragging down" pains in the abdomen during menses. During labour just one dose should be given initially and the patient's response carefully monitored. Never repeat the dose when it is still working or it will cause an aggravation of the pain. Also useful for retained placenta.

Caulophyllum 30c (blue cohosh) can also be given to bring on contractions if they have ceased.

Glenis (E-News)

Hemorrhage Rx

Look the woman directly in the eyes and tell her firmly to stop bleeding.

Judy Edmunds, WA

Collect a syringe full of the mother's hemorrhaged blood and insert the blood into the woman's anus. It is easily reabsorbed into her body. [Editor's Note: This was done in Japan in the early days of midwifery when there was no other recourse.]

Aki Otani, Osaka, Japan

Use press/release, press/release external stimulation of the uterus rather than tight holding.

Keep the mother warm. Shivering produces adrenaline, which in turn inhibits the production of oxytocin.

Ina May Gaskin, TN

Make a Heel Prick Easier

Use a capillary tube to draw up blood from a PKU heel prick (a blood test for phenylketonuria). It keeps blood from clotting when the wound is touched to the paper. It usually takes only three "draws" from one poke (the heel has been warmed) to complete.

Patricia Edmonds, OR

Newborn Care & Breastfeeding

Kangaroo Care: Why Does It Work?

by Holly Richardson

By THE EARLY 1980s, the mortality rate for premature infants in Bogota, Colombia, was 70 percent. The babies were dying of infections and respiratory problems, as well as lack of attention paid to them by a bonded parent. "Kangaroo care" for these infants evolved out of necessity. Mothers of premature infants were given their babies to hold 24 hours a day; they slept with them and tucked them under their clothing as if in a kangaroo's pouch. If a baby needed oxygen, it was administered under an oxygen hood placed on the mother's chest.

Doctors who conducted a concurrent study of this kangaroo care noticed a precipitous drop in neonatal mortality. Babies were not only surviving, they were thriving. Currently in Bogota, babies who are born as early as 10 weeks before their due date are going home within 24 hours! The criteria for these babies are that they be alive, able to breathe on their own, pink and able to suck. However, their weight is followed closely, and they can be gavage-fed if necessary.

Dr. Susan Ludington is one of the people who have been most instrumental in bringing kangaroo care to the United States. She has been intimately involved in many research projects, and her work is having a powerful, positive impact on premature babies and their families. In the United States, the few hospitals that regularly use kangaroo care protocols have mothers or fathers "wear" their babies for two to three hours per day, skin-to-skin. The baby is naked except for a diaper, and something must cover his or her back—either the parent's clothing or a receiving blanket folded in fourths. The baby is in a mostly upright position against the parent's chest.

The benefits of kangaroo care are numerous: The baby has a more stable heart rate (no bradycardia), more regular breathing (a 75 percent decrease in apneic episodes), improved oxygen saturation levels, no cold stress, longer periods of sleep, more rapid weight gain, more rapid brain development, reduction of "purposeless" activity, decreased crying, longer periods of alertness, more successful breastfeeding episodes, and earlier hospital discharge.

Benefits to the parents include "closure" over having a baby in a Neonatal Intensive Care Unit (NICU); feeling close to their babies (earlier bonding); having confidence that they can care for their baby, even better than hospital staff; gaining confidence that their baby is well cared for; and feeling in control—not to mention significantly decreased cost!

Why Does Kangaroo Care Work?
Why are Dr. Ludington and others seeing such phenomenal results with babies in kangaroo care? What is happening to the baby and the mother during this time?

One of the first things to happen is that maintenance of the baby's body temperature begins to depend on the mother, requiring the baby to use fewer calories to stay warm. Mothers naturally modulate the warmth of their breasts to keep their infants at the optimal temperature at which babies sleep best, have the best oxygen saturation levels, the least caloric expenditure and so forth. Maternal breast temperature can rise rapidly, then fall off as baby is warmed. As the baby starts to cool, the breasts heat up again—as much as 2°C in two minutes!

Being next to mom also helps the baby regulate his or her respiratory and heart rates. Babies experience significantly less bradycardia, and often none at all. The respiratory rate of kangarooed infants becomes more stable. The depth of each breath becomes more even, and apnea decreases fourfold and often disappears altogether. If apneic episodes do occur, the length of each episode decreases. In my own experience with a baby in NICU for bradycardia and apnea, I found that both problems disappeared completely when I was home kangarooing my baby.

During kangaroo care, a premature baby's overall growth rate increases. This is in part due to the baby's ability to sleep, thus conserving energy and putting caloric expenditure toward growth. According to Dr. Ludington, during the last six weeks of pregnancy, babies sleep 20 to 22 hours per day. In a typical NICU, however, they spend less than two hours total in deep, quiet sleep. Most of that comes in 10- or 20-second snatches. With kangaroo care, the infant typically snuggles into the breast and is deeply asleep within just a few minutes. These babies gain weight faster than their non-kangarooed counterparts, and it is interesting to note that they usually do not lose any of their birth weight.

Researchers have gained significant insight into what happens to an infant's brain during kangaroo care. Any baby's heart rate and respiratory rates can be plotted as a sort of artistic drawing. Because premature infants lack the ability to coordinate their breathing and heart rates, the rates "plot out" as chaotic. This means with increased demand on the cardiovascular system, as with crying or fussing, the system does not respond with a related increase in cardiac output. In other words, the baby's respiratory rate may increase while crying, but the heart rate does not. As premies mature, these rates become synchronized, or "coupled," resulting in an orderly drawing when the rates are plotted together. The drawing no longer looks random.

In infants in kangaroo care, researchers found that coupling takes place after only 10 minutes. This hardly seemed possible because it equaled four weeks of brain development in the "normal" premie. As researchers studied brain wave

(Continued on next page)

patterns of infants in kangaroo care, they found two significant things. First, there was a doubling of alpha waves—the brain wave pattern associated with contentment and bliss. Second, they found that "delta brushes" were occurring. Delta brushes happen only when new synapses are being formed. So holding the infant skin-to-skin allows his or her brain to continue its work of developing neural synapses.

Imagine the implications if all infants "at risk" were kangarooed. Dr. Ludington sums up kangaroo care very aptly by saying, "Separation is not biologically normal."

Helping our clients understand their options, including risks, benefits and alternatives, is a very important part of being "with woman." Knowing enough about kangaroo care to help them make informed decisions is another important tool for the caregiver's birth bag. All infants benefit from skin-to-skin contact, breastfeeding, shared sleep and so forth, but some babies very seriously need kangaroo care, They include premature infants, infants with low muscle tone or disabilities, high-needs infants, those with intrauterine growth retardation or those who have a hard time gaining weight. Midwives would do well to learn the basics of kangaroo care and where to turn for further information. Adding Dr. Ludington's book *Kangaroo Care* to one's library is a good first step. Being supportive of parents and giving encouragement and positive reinforcement are also very helpful. Remember that in some instances, kangaroo care has meant the difference between life and death.

References

Ludington-Hoe, S.M. and Golant, S.K. (1993). *Kangaroo Care: The Best You Can Do for Your Premature Infant.* New York: Bantam Books.

Ludington, S.M. (1997). Conference presentation, with mention of research in progress.

Ludington, S.M. Kangaroo Care Bibliography. Current to March 1997.

Cuddle Up! Slings and Baby Carriers

by Jennifer Rosenberg

I'D ALWAYS ASSUMED I'd use some sort of baby carrier, but when I got pregnant, I was familiar with only the Snuggli front packs. My mom had used one with my sister. My midwife told me there were other ways of carrying a baby and introduced me to the Baby Bundler, which was my daughter's first carrier. I did not own a stroller until she was 2 months old, and even then, with the bus as my sole transportation, the stroller was too unwieldy for me to use most of the time.

The Bundler made possible shopping and nursing at the same time, and it simplified my life dramatically. I became more interested in baby-wearing and was introduced to the New Native Baby Carrier when Kailea was 10 months old. It was perfect for her "up-down" phase, since I could wear it around the house with or without a baby in it. The design was simple enough that I made several slings in the same shape but out of different fabrics; it was a rare day I didn't have my daughter on my hip.

I made some slings for friends and for my clients as a doula. When I returned to working on a regular basis, I stopped sewing, but the numerous slings out there still fascinated me, and I became more interested in the many ways non-Western cultures wear their babies. It frustrated me that I hadn't been taught how to make a sling or carrier out of the materials at hand. Not until I was helping a young mom with a 1-month-old, high-needs baby did I start to recapture some of that knowledge. While I cleaned for her, I listened to her frustration about living on Ramen noodles during the day because it was the only food she could make with one hand, having a baby who wanted to be held constantly.

I mentioned slings, and she spoke of a dream she'd had in which she'd tied her baby to her with a sheet. She explained how it had worked in the dream, and in a flash of inspiration, I said, "But you wouldn't do it like that, you'd do it folded."

I folded it twice and wrapped it around her, tied it in a square knot, and slipped her baby into the cozy pocket the folds had made. She laughed with relief, and said, "Now I can make a peanut butter and jelly sandwich! I have two hands free!"

Here was a sling that was cheap (almost free, since everyone has bed sheets), easy to use and easy to demonstrate. It was a little bulky, not the prettiest sling in the world, not a long-term solution, but wonderful for making life easier in the short term. No sewing was required, and the "sling" could easily become a sheet again. I still preferred my tube sling for ease of use, but what a relief to be able to provide a sling on the spot.

I wanted to share this concept with as many midwives, doulas and moms as possible so that we could reclaim baby-wearing as an easy thing, not an exotic or expensive thing. At that point I didn't know much about rebozos, or different kinds of carriers and slings—just the few I'd tried. I took my idea to a Tricks of the Trade circle at

Midwifery Today's Eugene '96 conference, and brought my 25-year-old sheet into the middle of the circle to demonstrate this to the midwives. Fusako Sei, a midwife from Japan, stepped forward, pulling a mom and babe out of the audience, and demonstrated a traditional Japanese-style carrier using the same sheet I'd used. Then the Inuit midwives showed us a variation of that carrier. At that point the mom asked me if she could have my sheet because it was so comfortable. Then one of the Mexican midwives brought out her rebozo and showed us a variety of carriers, some similar to the one I'd done and others very different. It was a cascade of shared knowledge that quenched my thirst for this fundamental information.

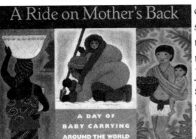

I've since read a precious book called *A Ride on Mother's Back*, which is a children's book about slings around the world. It's beautiful and shows the many ways of wearing a babe. I feel strongly that every mother should know how to wear her baby, whether or not she chooses to use that knowledge. How many times have you seen a mother at a bus stop juggling a stroller, baby, diaper bag and a toddler? How many times have you seen a parent with weary arms lugging a 30-pound toddler through a mall, carrying the child because his little legs got tired?

As birth professionals we should know these techniques and pass them on to our clients. We are in a unique position to influence our clients, and this particular information can have far-reaching effects on the quality of their lives. Let's reclaim the wisdom of carrying our babies.

Techniques for Making Slings

Take any flat sheet larger than a crib sheet and smaller than a king-sized sheet. Fold it lengthwise and then fold it lengthwise again. At this point you will have a long strip of fabric. Find the middle of the length. Place the thickest fold "down" on the hip of the person who will wear the sling. Bring one end of the folded sheet up behind the person's back and over the person's opposite shoulder. Bring the other end up in front of her, across her body, then tie the two ends of the fabric in front of the shoulder, so that the knot is in front of the shoulder, and the fabric is spread out across the shoulder and across the back.

Don't tie the sling too tightly—leave a bit of play, which can be snugged up after the baby is in the sling. This creates a pocket in the sheet, into which the baby will be put. Hold the baby on one shoulder with one hand. With the other hand, pull apart two of the layers of the sling, and guide the baby's feet in between. Holding the sling open, use the other hand to allow the baby to slide down slowly into the sling pocket.

Newborns will snuggle into a ball between mother's breasts. They can be adjusted a bit so that the knot on the fabric helps to support the head. A rolled up washcloth also works well to support the head. Older babies will go more off center, toward the hip, and may want to be looking out more. They can sit in the sling facing mom or facing out. Once baby is in place, the knot can be loosened slightly, and the sling can be snugged so that the baby stays easily in place and mom feels secure.

Once a good fit is achieved, it is unnecessary in most cases to repeatedly tie and untie the sling, as it can be simply slipped off over the head and slipped back on the same way. If the fabric slips, it can be pinned with diaper pins or sewn in place once a good fit is achieved. I find that once the sling is tightened, it doesn't slip if a square knot is used. If desired, for a lighter weight sling, a twin or queen sheet may be cut in half lengthwise and hemmed down the cut edge. This will need to be folded only once. It makes two slings.

(Continued on next page)

Sling Ideas

1. Make tube-slings out of birdseye fabric (cheap, sturdy, cotton diaper fabric, not flannel). Donate them to your local NICU or labor and delivery ward. Cost: $3 to $6 per sling. Time: 10-30 minutes per sling.
2. Buy bed sheets at Goodwill, the Salvation Army or other thrift stores. Cut them in half, serge or hem the raw edges, wash them, and then use them as slings you can give away if you see tired moms in the mall or grocery store hip-carrying a toddler or baby. Give them your business card at the same time. Cost: about 35 cents to 50 cents per sling. Time: 5-30 minutes per sling. (Overlock sewing machines make this task completely simple.)
3. Make your clients tube-style slings out of cotton interlock as a birth gift. Or add the cost of fabric onto your fee if they want a sling. Cost: $4 to $15 per sling. Time: 30-40 minutes per sling, including fitting. If you want to get fancy, get or make labels with your name, practice name and phone number on them, and sew them onto each sling. This is great advertising, both for baby wearing and for midwifery/doula services.
4. If you don't sew, or don't have time for sewing, ask your apprentice to do it, or see if you can find a sewing circle or church group that would like to donate their skills to making slings for low-income moms. The "bed sheet" style slings using recycled sheets make a wonderfully easy gift for new moms.

Tips & Tricks

Diaper Wipes

One of my babies had famously delicate skin, sensitive to everything, and I didn't dare use packaged diaper wipes on him. In an old health care book, I discovered a recipe for oil soap:

Mix about a cup of almond or other stable, good-quality oil with several tablespoons of anhydrous lanolin. An egg whip works well to mix them. You can also use vegetable shortening or even zinc oxide cream as the thickener; the amount is determined by how thick you want the mixture to be. Calendula oil or tincture, or other skin-friendly herbal oils or tinctures, can be added. Put the mixture in a bottle with a strong flip top, and use like diaper wipes, pouring as much as is needed on a soft cloth or tissue. It cleans well, no rinsing is needed, and it leaves the skin soft.

Gail Hart, America Online

Natural Baby Wipes

2 cups warm purified water
1-1/2 tsp. natural plain castile soap
1-1/2 tsp. natural baby oil or lotion
60 "Job Squad" half towels
Mix liquids together, then pour over towels a few at a time. Store in an airtight container.

Oklahoma Midwives Assn., Tulsa, OK

Colic Solutions

Cinnamon tea, best made by stirring a cinnamon stick in hot water for 10 seconds and given by dropperful, can ease colic.

I have seen much success with pantothenic acid. Crush one tablet (100mg) and mix with water. Give this to baby around the same time every day. The baby will probably ingest half the solution (50mg), which is just about right. It takes a few days to start working, but parents swear by it.

Rain Taylor, DEM, CA

These sheets also make excellent hip carriers. To make a hip carrier out of a length of fabric, simply tie it in a sash, with the knot in front of the shoulder, and set the baby on the bottom of the sash on the hip.

A long strip of fabric can be turned into a back carrier by placing the middle of the fabric behind the child's back and bringing the fabric under the child's arms. The child is then placed high on the parent's back, with the parent leaning forward a bit. (There's a knack to this that involves keeping a hold on the fabric while swinging the child around to the back, then using the fabric to hold the child in place while the sling is finished.) The ends of the fabric come over the parent's shoulders, cross in front across the parent's chest, and then wrap around behind the parent, over the child's legs, and tie under the child's bottom in the middle of the parent's back. This allows both the child's and parent's arms to be free. This is a comfortable carrier and does not displace the parent's center of gravity to the same degree as a backpack does. This is a comfortable way to carry a walking child who is a bit too heavy to carry in a sling for extended periods of time.

The same theory can be used to make a warmer back-carry that's good for both toddlers and babies as young as about 3 months. Instead of a long strip of fabric, a very large triangle is used, and the child's arms may either be free or trapped by the fabric. The knot secures the "point" of the triangle, making a large shawl for the baby and mother. The general placement and technique are similar. The baby rides fairly high up while the carrier is being tied, then slips down a little once the knot is in place. A rebozo (a very large woven scarf) can be slung over one shoulder and tied at the opposite hip to tie a baby on, similar to the bed sheet sling. Or it can be folded and tied in front of the shoulder.

There are many other ways of wearing babies; these are the ones I know and share with you. If you have other ways, I would love to hear of them. Please send them to me, in care of Midwifery Today, along with any pictures. My goal is to teach as many people as possible the different ways of holding and carrying babies so that mothers will have an easier time of caring for their little ones, and their little ones will have an easier time growing up.

I see slings as basic items of clothing, and I recommend that my clients have several available, try different kinds, and wear their babies as often as they can. Each sling, carrier, backpack and hip carrier has its place and appeal. One mom who wouldn't think of using a fabric sling loved the high-tech fanny pack I got from the Cuddle Karrier company. It converts into a sling-like carrier but goes back to being a fanny pack easily. Just as different styles of parenting work for different people, there are different carriers that work for different mothers. As long as the baby is being carried, that's the whole point.

Milk Angels

by Jennifer Rosenberg

VIA MY COMPUTER, I speak with many women around the world who plan to breastfeed, try to breastfeed and then struggle with breastfeeding until they wean to formula. The most common barrier to successful nursing for these women seems to be a lack of support at critical times.

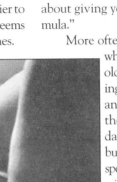

photo by Judith Halek

We've known for years that the strongest predictor of nursing success is good advice and support for breastfeeding moms. Today we have more resources, more knowledge and more support for breastfeeding than we've had for years, such as lactation consultants and the La Leche League.

Why isn't this enough? I believe the problem is simple: babies' needs can't be scheduled.

Many moms tell me, "I got great help in the hospital, but once I got home, everything fell apart"; or "I had my baby on the weekend, and the hospital's lactation consultant works only on weekdays"; or "The lactation consultant can see me tomorrow at 2 o'clock in the afternoon, but my baby is hungry now and I can't get her latched on!"

As a doula, I'm comfortable with the concept of being on call. If a client goes into labor, I can't tell her, "I'm sorry, I have room for you in my schedule tomorrow morning at 10." I don't expect her to put up with her contractions knowing help will be there tomorrow. Tomorrow may be too late.

We need a similar approach when it comes to the first weeks of breastfeeding. I tell my nursing mothers, "I want you to call if nursing hurts, I want you to call if you're getting frustrated, and I want you to call if you're even thinking about giving your baby a bottle of formula."

More often than not, I call them when their baby is a few days old and ask them how nursing is going. If they indicate any problems at all, I go to them—not the following day, not three hours later, but within the hour. I rarely spend more than a half-hour with them at their houses.

When I go sit with them and watch them struggle to nurse, I usually need only help make a small adjustment: pull a lip here, place a hand there, calm the baby down, calm the mom down. Small things. The baby will latch, and the mom will see it can be done. This might happen at 11 o'clock in the morning, but just as often it happens at 10 at night. If it happens during the day, I call a few hours later and ask how it is going. If it happened at night, I call the next morning. I always get one of two answers: either everything is fine (in which case I will call back the next day just to make sure), or there is still a problem. Sometimes I refer my clients to lactation consultants; other times I simply get back in my car and go sit with them.

One client had a baby who would only latch on well when I was there. So I told the mom if she had to call me 18 times in the next 24 hours to get it to work, that would be fine with me. I took the pressure off her—gave her permission to ask for help. We discussed strategies, options, talked about her alternatives. She called two or three times. I called her a couple of times to check in with her. Two days later, her answer to "How is nursing going?" was "Just fine! No problems!" She's still nursing her daughter several months later.

Tips & Tricks

A Calming Bath
To help soothe a colicky or fussy baby, have mom get into a warm bath with the baby. Floating will calm him.

Tricks of the Trade Circle, NY '94

Leave the Vernix On
I stumbled on an interesting article in an old British OB-GYN journal; it indicated that vernix should be left on a newborn rather than washed off because it assists the infant in maintaining body temperature. Forget the newborn bath!

Phylis Austin, GA

No Hurry, No Worry
I give my clients the following advice: bathe the baby whenever they wish. There is no need to hurry and no need to delay. Bathing before the cord detaches does no harm and does not increase the incidence of infection.

Gail Hart (E-News)

Leave Cord Stumps Alone
For the last year or so I haven't put anything on umbilical cord stumps and tell parents to do what they feel is best. I have noticed that the time it takes for the cord stump to fall off has decreased remarkably since I stopped having parents use alcohol to clean the stump.

Margie Dacko, NV

Empathy Needed
Baby has never known sight, smell, touch, temperature regulation, hunger, voiding, or night and day as we know them. All baby's needs were met on a constant basis before birth. Understanding this makes it easier to help baby adjust to its new environment. For example, babies like to be swaddled. Some also prefer motion (which explains why baby wakes up when an expectant mom lies down to rest!). Perfume and other strong smells can upset them. Reminding the new mother about these things may make her transition into motherhood a little easier.

Rain Taylor, DEM, CA

We have an extraordinary pool of talent and resources to draw on right now. We have doulas, La Leche League, lactation consultants, midwives, childbirth
(Continued on next page)

educators, nurses and postpartum doulas. We have telephones, pagers, e-mail and the Internet. We also have a growing foundation of scientific and practical knowledge about breastfeeding.

Every woman who wants to nurse her baby should have all the support she needs to do so successfully. But these resources are not being utilized, and in many areas, the resources are not available.

My dream is that a mother learning to nurse her baby will be able to pick up her phone, call someone knowledgeable, talk about what is going on with her and her baby, and have a "milk angel" sitting on her couch to help her through any crisis within 45 minutes. It would be a form of triage.

I am in favor of an on-call crisis breastfeeding support service that would be offered by doulas, experienced moms and La Leche League leaders. For the majority of women, a half-hour or hour of assistance will be all that is necessary—as long as it is provided when it is needed. When that crisis visit does not solve the problem, a visit with a lactation consultant would be scheduled for more intensive help.

Think about it. Instead of moms giving babies bottles out of frustration and panic because their screaming baby can't wait until tomorrow morning at 10 o'clock to get help latching on, moms would know help is 45 minutes, not 15 hours away. The milk angel can help them find alternatives to bottles so that the baby does not have nipple confusion to contend with as well.

I am not a lactation consultant. When I do breastfeeding support, I do basic things, like untucking the bottom lip, correcting the position of the hand on the breast, getting the baby to latch on quickly to my finger without chewing before the mom puts the baby to her tender nipple.

Sometimes when I first walk in, if the mom and baby are both frantic and there is milk expressed already, I will show the mom how to use a spoon or small cup to drip the milk into the baby's mouth. This calms the baby down and soothes the mother's fear that her baby isn't getting anything to eat.

I don't set moms up with breast pumps or nipple shields or supplemental nutrition systems (SNS). I don't do intensive suck training or teach them how to finger feed. I always refer moms with inverted nipples and babies with weak sucks.

Perhaps the most important thing I do is respond quickly and go to the clients, rather than making the clients come to me or schedule an appointment. I know that if I go right away, I'll only have to take a half-hour or an hour of my time to help them. If I wait, we may have a much longer row to hoe.

Say I didn't go to my client at 10:30 at night—what would she do? Tough it out? Send her husband to the store to buy formula and bottles? But then the mom may have to use a breast pump to get her supply back up. She may be engorged. She may get a breast infection. She may not go to the lactation consultant at all, but simply wean to formula and bottles because her baby stopped screaming and drank four ounces and slept through the night. Maybe she nurses through the pain of a bad latch for months. If she has suffered through any of these possible scenarios, she remembers those first months as a time of pain, a time of failure and a time of crisis. I'd rather she be able to enjoy nursing, feel the success of a baby who doubles her birth weight in her first two to three months, feel the pleasure of nursing when it doesn't hurt, and experience the wonder of a baby falling asleep on her breast, completely content.

Money

Ideally, grants, insurance companies, doctors and hospitals would fund a program such as the "Milk Angels." It should be part of standard care. Another option would be to have clients of the program pay on a sliding scale, ranging from $5 to $30 per visit. Realistically, given the skill level and time involved in an average visit, $15-$20 would be a reasonable reimbursement for a milk angel for a single 30-60 minute home visit with phone follow-up. I base this on the average hourly rate that childbirth educators and doulas make per hour ($10-$20), and considering that each visit may require child care, driving time and being on-call. As a doula, I do many of these visits for free because I feel it is so important for women to get the help they need. Many of my clients tip me substantially, which makes up for those who cannot afford to pay me extra for milk angel visits.

Given the fact that lactation consultants often charge between $45 and $60 per visit, this seems very reasonable and a good way to help families feel that if they do end up hiring a lactation consultant, it is really necessary to have someone with that level of training to help.

Messages Moms Need to Hear

1. You can do this!
2. It gets better.
3. Your baby is learning with you. It's not your fault.
4. In the next couple of days it will get much easier.
5. When we figure this out, it will probably get better quicker than you think is possible.

A Model for Ideal Breastfeeding Support

1. From the beginning, moms need good help getting the baby latched on.
2. When the milk comes in, it is important that someone touch base with moms to make sure they are doing well emotionally and that nursing is going well.
3. If nursing is not going well on the second or third day (when someone checks in with the mom via phone), a milk angel will be sent to observe the mom breastfeed and provide basic assistance.
4. Breastfeeding help via phone should be available 24 hours per day. If phone help is not enough, a milk angel should be sent to help the mom in her home.
5. Lactation consultants should be available for more intensive help in more complicated cases.
6. Breastfeeding support groups, such as La Leche League, and peer support programs should be available for all women who want them.

Breast Yeast

by Chris Hafner-Eaton, PhD

IT'S BEEN A particularly rainy year in the Pacific Northwest and as the Oregon La Leche League Area professional liaison, I've received numerous calls regarding "incurable sore nipples" and breast pain. What do these two things have to do with each other and the provocative title?

In many cases so-called incurable sore nipples and phantom deep breast pain are neither incurable nor phantom, but rather are caused by an undiagnosed yeast overgrowth. Ubiquitous yeast, also known as thrush or Candidiasis, has a synergistic or compound relationship with other fungus or molds that increase during damp, rainy weather. As for the title, thrush often looks like cotton in the mouth, and one over-the-counter treatment (gentian violet) results in a very purple-mouthed child whom my 5-year-old thinks is funny. While as lay support persons we do not diagnose medical conditions, we are often called upon once the medical community has "given up" on a particular case—that is, mother and baby have been handed formula. Thus, if a mother has been told there's nothing wrong with her by a physician/nurse/other health professional, yet she is in excruciating pain or her baby clearly is suffering, she may seek out nonmedical support. Older literature sources document that health care professionals often overlook breast yeast.

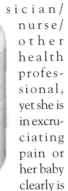

To help mothers identify possible underlying causes of pain, lay support persons should thoroughly examine a pregnant mom's histories of pregnancy, labor and delivery, as well as her nursing experience to date. Of course, latch-on should be verified and corrected, and if possible checked in person. Yeast red flags, as I call them, include: any procedure that typically requires antibiotics after delivery, such as c-section or tubal ligation, corticosteroid use (terbutaline to delay labor, or asthma medications), prednisone for allergic reactions, any other immune suppression (such as being HIV positive), diabetes, or even long-term use of histamine blockers such as Seldane. Other less clear clues range from cravings of sugars and breads to extreme fatigue.

Moms describe the classic symptoms of breast yeast in various ways (these are eloquently described in the La Leche League International Lactation Series No. 18). These symptoms include: severe pain without nipple trauma; sharp, shooting pains radiating from nipple—may extend to chest wall or back; nipples that may be red, flaky, itchy, shiny or burning (ask the mother what is normal for her); small white, hard blisters on the nipple (may also be blocked pores); or sometimes white fuzzy patches in the folds of the nipple. When moms describe nursing as an "ice pick" or "glass" inside their breast, or pain that persists beyond latch-on, yeast overgrowth in the milk ducts may be the cause.

Breast yeast frequently does not have visible symptoms, but, as one author describes, it is "exquisitely painful." Low-level thrush also may not have visible signs. Nursing may be going well, and all of the sudden it hurts or the baby is pulling off the breast (sometimes baby makes a clicking or popping sound). In most cases if the latch has been assessed and/or corrected, the offending agent is Candida albicans, but there are several other strains of candida and not all of them grow fluffy patches of cotton, the usual harbinger of yeast or thrush. As a public health professional, I have seen several other agents of fungus overgrowth—aspergillus and a few found usually in the garden. These are much less likely causes of nipple and breast pain; however, they are possible, and practitioners should be aware of them.

Over-the-counter and self-help approaches to yeast management can be quite effective, particularly if they are part of a comprehensive, holistic approach to this problem and if the problem hasn't become chronic. Because this tactic is holistic, I believe it is appropriate for us to present this information as an option to mothers dealing with yeast. Empowered and informed mothers can then decide for themselves what to do. With a few caveats, there are no negative effects to this approach. As with many health conditions, it is helpful for both the support person and mother to understand why yeast overgrowth occurs so that they aren't simply chasing symptoms.

First understand that yeasts love dark, moist, warm places (think of how bread rises). They also thrive in sweet environments, and they multiply faster than proverbial rabbits. These factors account for why diabetics and pregnant and lactating women are all prime candidates for yeast overgrowth. If you have ever added into the mix any immunosuppression of the natural forces that keep your body in balance—such as broad-spectrum antibiotics or corticosteroids, especially taken within the past few months—the yeasts may grow unchecked. Along with the common recommendations of changing breast pads at each feeding, going bra-less and applying topical treatments, it is essential to deal with the underlying health status of the mother and baby, and sometimes the entire family. This means that regardless of the type of treatment—prescription, naturopathic, homeopathic or other—we need to also address certain issues such as hygiene, diet and laundry.

In a nursing relationship it is imperative that both the mother
(Continued on next page)

and the baby be treated, even if only one is symptomatic. Many times the father and siblings require lower-level treatment as well. In co-sleeping arrangements all members who sleep in close contact should be treated. A particularly frustrating aspect of yeast management stems from the fact that treatment needs to be continued for two weeks after symptoms subside.

Personal hygiene is also very important in yeast control. While antibacterial soaps are promoted for new parents, they may actually contribute to yeast overgrowth by killing the "good" bacteria. Still, hands do need to be washed with warm water and soap after diaper changes and using the bathroom. In addition, short-term switching to paper towels (used only once) as a drying method can help stop fungal spread. Temporary use of disposable diapers may help too. A spray bottle of vinegar solution (1/4 cup white vinegar to one cup of water) should be available for all family members to spray any areas on their bodies that stay or get moist (pubic areas, armpits, under breasts and under any folds of skin). This routine should be used at least twice a day by those not symptomatic and four times per day by those with symptoms and continued for two weeks beyond the time anyone shows symptoms.

Bath towels should not be shared, and they ideally should be used only once. If that seems extreme, then the towels must be allowed to dry thoroughly after each use. In addition, items such as toothbrushes and makeup can also harbor yeast spores. Once the anti-yeast regimen is begun, every family member should get new toothbrushes and then again once all symptoms disappear. No cornstarch powders or deodorants should be used, as they are a food source for yeast. As for makeup, as expensive as it is, one might try not wearing it during the early treatment time, then dispose of all makeup and buy new supplies. Since the eyelids have folds and the mouth may harbor yeast, the minimum would be to replace eye-liner, shadows, mascara, lipstick/pencils and foundations, as well as any applicators that cannot be treated.

Household treatment clearly means more work—not something relished by new mothers—but it still must occur for chronic cases to be cleared. This means that sources of mold—wet window sills, damp laundry hampers, and bathtubs (especially the jetted kind)—need to be cleaned with either a 10 percent bleach solution or white vinegar in water. Floors, baseboards and walls may all be cleaned by the same method. Laundry should be washed in the hottest possible water and a cup of white distilled vinegar added to the final rinse. Relying on bleach in the washer is not sufficient, since it would take a gallon of bleach in a standard washer to kill yeast spores and would result in Swiss cheese clothing. Boiling clothing and other items of close contact (such as underwear and sheets) for five minutes will work, as will microwaving on high for five minutes.

Freezing will not kill yeast spores. Cloth diapers, either from a service or your own, should also be microwaved for five minutes on high. Toys and any items babies mouth or chew should also be cleaned this way. They may be put in the dishwasher if your water is hot enough (over 130 degrees) and you add vinegar to the rinse. (I strongly suggest enlisting help for all these matters so that the mother can get needed rest.)

In addition to the hygiene and household measures described and the dietary recommendations in the references listed, a number of naturopathic treatments are available for mothers. The range of naturopathic treatments used for yeast includes: acidophilus, vinegar, baking soda, garlic capsules, nonyeast-based B complex, zinc, vitamin C, caprylic acid, citrus seed oil, tea tree oil, Pau D'arco, echinacea, maitake tea, heparsulfur and gentian violet (use with caution).

The following is a very brief alphabetized overview of how to utilize these in the case of breast yeast. For more detailed information on their general use, see the sources listed.

Acidophilus (*Lactobacillus acidophilus*): work up to three capsules three times daily; babies may be treated with diluted acidophilus in breastmilk swabbed or dropped into their mouths, or mom may dip a finger in the powder and let baby suck. It may also be applied to breast and diaper areas directly. The intent of acidophilus treatment is to rebalance the body, so don't expect instant results. Yogurt made with live cultures also has a therapeutic effect, but is considerably slower.

Tips & Tricks
Colic Remedies

Catnip and fennel tincture is a favorite; use a few drops in a little water, as needed.

Italian grandmothers all recommend bay leaf tea. Steep a few bay leaves (right from your spice shelf) in water. I have seen this work; it often results in a good loud burp, and a much happier baby!

Massage can help. I recommend a class or at least a book that covers the basics. The most important thing to remember is to rub upward on the right side of the tummy and down on the left. This stroke follows the large intestine and helps move gas in the best direction for getting relief. Using a light, warmed vegetable oil often makes this very comforting. I enjoy using cocoa butter.

Bicycling the baby's legs often helps the baby to pass gas.

Some hypertonic babies overstimulate readily. For them, caution is needed where touch and other stimulation are concerned. This type of baby benefits from swaddling and a stable and somewhat quiet environment.

Rain Taylor, DEM, CA

Used in conjunction with the capsules, and even as a soothing breast paste, yogurt can help rebalance the body; however, it is unlikely that acute cases will be cleared with this method alone. Sometimes lactobacilli need a bit of help getting hold in the intestines, and some practitioners recommend FOS (fructo-oligo-saccharides) to enhance colonization.

B Complex: a set of strong immune system boosters that may be lacking in the mother's and baby's intestines if they have had antibiotics. B complex (100 mg each of each B vitamin) is water-soluble and needs to be time released or taken throughout the day in three doses. It may turn breastmilk (as well as urine) yellow.

Baking Soda: make a paste in water and swab the baby's mouth after each feeding (if baby always falls asleep, then do it whenever possible, but at least four times per day).

Barberry (*Berberis vulgaris*): consume three times a day either 1-2 grams dried bark, or 1.5 tsp. (4-6 ml) of tincture (1:5), or 250-500 mg of powdered extract.

Caprylic Acid: a strong antifungal taken orally; two to three capsules three to four times per day for two weeks (or 1 gram at meals). These capsules must be enterically coated so that they release their active ingredients in the intestines.

Citrus Seed Oil: a strong but natural antifungal, antibacterial and antiviral. May be used topically but must be diluted before use on breast or on any mucous membrane. Try 10 drops in one-quarter cup water swallowed at once, twice daily

Garlic: although increasing dietary garlic may be useful, clinically effective doses are easier to get if you take triple strength deodorized garlic tablets (three tablets, three times daily for two weeks or more). The liquid, cold pressed, aged garlic is thought to be most potent. Kyolic is the brand from which the most conclusive research was published. These may cause gas, although some researchers believe this is a sign that the yeast is dying off in the intestines. Contrary to old myths, garlic has been shown to increase the amount of breastmilk babies consume. Note: ginger and cinnamon also have reported antifungal activity, but their use is infrequently reported and primarily unstudied.

Gentian Violet: one of the oldest (preceding topical iodine) antifungal antiseptics available is still an over-the-counter and inexpensive method available (less than $2.) It is very effective and extremely messy, staining everything that comes in its path. Gentian violet should be used only for a maximum of 2-3 days (two treatments per day) by coating the nipple, areola and surrounding breast tissue with the liquid on a cotton ball. The long-term toxicity of this treatment is still being debated, but short-term treatment appears to cause no ill effects. Still, this is a treatment of latter resort as an over-the-counter method because of the mess. Nursing babies will get a purple mouth, which will wear off in a few days. Suggest that the mother wear clothing that can be thrown away or bleached.

Goldenseal Powder: (CAUTION) Although very bitter, this herb is very effective at clearing yeast from the body Make a tea using one-half teaspoon goldenseal per cup of boiling water and drink throughout the day. Susan Weed (see references) suggests this as a last resort because it kills the beneficial bacteria in the intestines and may cause diarrhea and colic.

Hydrastis Candadensis: Consume three times a day either 1-2 grams dried bark or 1.5 tsp. (4-6 ml) of tincture (1:5), or 250-500 mg of powdered extract.

Ibuprofen: an over-the-counter anti-inflammatory that might be appropriate for both pain relief and reducing ductile inflammation. If the mother is in tremendous pain, an anti-inflammatory may help until proper treatment addresses the cause. (Acetaminophen does not address the inflammation.) Of course, the baby's reactions should be closely monitored with any treatment.

Maitake Tea: an antifungal tea that also helps to rebalance intestinal flora. Drink several cups per day at the strongest possible brew.

Massage and Warm Compresses: compresses should be soaked either with vinegar and water or with olive oil. In addition, deeply massage out any possible plugged ducts with arnica oil as a lubricant. Massage while baby nurses, taking advantage of gravity if possible.

Olive Oil: apply topically to breasts after each feeding. Olive oil contains linoleic acids, which are antifungal.

Pau D'arco (*Tabebuiaimpetiginosa*): an antifungal tincture with a long history of use in developing countries. It tastes horrible and must be taken four times a day (20-30 drops).

Plantain Seeds (*Plantago major*): soak seeds overnight in warm water, then apply the resultant gel topically and/or orally.

Potassium Sorbate: one Tbsp. dissolved in one quart warm water applied topically. This product is commonly used to stop fermentation and is available at wine-making supply stores and pharmacies.

Tea Tree Oil: an Australian antiseptic oil thought to have antifungal properties. A few drops may be added to bath water or diluted and applied to breast. The bath method may be used with vinegar and has the added benefit of helping clear the sinuses.

Vaginal Yeast Creams: (over-the-counter) with Miconazole or Clotrimazole: some practitioners
(Continued on next page)

have started suggesting these be used for breast yeast. While they may be effective and the active ingredients are compatible with nursing, there may be other ingredients not appropriate for babies to consume. Use this approach with caution (perhaps rinsing the cream off before nursing).

Vinegar: start with one-quarter cup white vinegar in 1 cup water. If this is too strong, mix a dilution as weak as one tablespoon in one cup of water and apply it topically to the breast. Allow to air dry. Do not wash it off before nursing unless baby protests. This must be done at least four times a day and maintained for two weeks after all symptoms are gone. Families may take baths with vinegar in the water to hit more than one source at a time. White distilled vinegar must be used because it has been boiled and has no active spores. Arguments about the logic of using vinegar (which is fermented) abound, but yeast cannot survive in the pH created by this and the temperature needed to distill it. And many mothers have found this works quite well when used with acidophilus to rebalance the intestines—if they catch the overgrowth early.

Vitamin C: up to the point where loose stools occur, then back off the dosage a bit. Since vitamin C is water-soluble it must be consumed throughout the day. Echinacea capsules or tincture can be taken simultaneously to boost the immune system.

Zinc: another immune system booster: 45mg per day.

If all this seems like a fanatical effort to eliminate yeast, it may be, but yeasts are extremely persistent in the right environment. If this isn't a reasonable course of action and/or you are working with a practitioner who believes pharmaceutical treatment should be used in conjunction, then some of the following information may be helpful. Unfortunately, moms often report not being able to find a practitioner willing to work with them on mixing pharmaceuticals and natural remedies. Also, lay support must be aware that yeast may co-exist with bacteria and that it is possible to have either yeast/fungal mastitis or bacterial mastitis coupled with yeast.

If the mother reports any symptoms of bacterial mastitis (fever of more than 102 degrees, flu-like symptoms, red streaks on the breast, hot spots on the breast, etc.) she should seek medical attention immediately, get lots of rest and nurse lying down. If yeast and bacteria are joint causes, in addition to taking antibiotics the mom may want to request oral Nystatin tablets to take along with the antibiotics.

Treatments Prescribed by Licensed Practitioners

If a health care provider is involved, the first usual line of defense prescribed for yeast is Nystatin (either cream or suspension). Nystatin is an exceptionally safe pharmaceutical that acts by disrupting the necessary enzymes yeasts need to reproduce, but it doesn't interfere with our systems. However, its effectiveness in killing yeast may cause side effects (nausea, gas and fatigue) as the yeasts die off. Nystatin must be religiously applied after every nursing, since yeast multiplies rapidly. Some researchers believe that Nystatin is not very effective because it is mixed in a sucrose base (in which yeast thrive); instead, they recommend using Nystatin powder mixed in water or other liquids (breast milk for babies).

If Nystatin is not effective initially, or the yeast becomes chronic or invades the ducts of the breast, other methods are available. Mycelia troches are often prescribed for the nursing pair. These tablets are crushed, mixed with breastmilk, and applied to thrush. Older babies may like chewing on the troches directly. The active ingredient is miconazole, which is also the ingredient in many over-the-counter vaginal yeast medications. If applied to the breast, the drug will be taken into the baby's mouth as would any topical that is not washed off. As a third line of defense in the topical war against yeast, some practitioners may resort to Nizoral 2% cream for the breast and diaper areas (Ketoconazole is the active ingredient).

Nizoral is also available systemically, although its effects on infants have not been studied. Nizoral tablets are a potent chemical whose side effects should be weighed against the possible benefits. Lastly, a new and now commonly prescribed vaginal yeast treatment, Diflucan (fluconazole), is being used to treat breast yeast. One dosage is used in cases of vaginal yeast, but experience has shown that breast yeast requires many more doses to fully clear the overgrowth. Diflucan has few side effects, is taken once per day, and is quite effective if given for a long enough period (usually 2-4 weeks—not one or two days) while the baby's mouth is simultaneously treated with another anti-yeast treatment. One should be

(Continued on next page)

Induced Lactation

Induced lactation often requires supplemental feeds which can be provided at the breast with a Supplemental Nursing system (SNS). Because they are overpriced, I make my own for clients who are on limited incomes. Take a No. 5 feeding tube and push it through a nipple (with appropriately sized hole.) Attach the nipple to a bottle in which there is formula. Place the bottle on a table or high enough to allow easy flow of the liquid to the baby—usually at the height of the baby's head. Tape the end of the feeding tube to the breast (do not use heavy tape—it hurts when removed!) allowing the end of the feeding tube to come to the end of the nipple or slightly beyond.

The advantages of this method of supplementation include nipple stimulation to increase maternal milk production while simultaneously providing baby with required nutrient and maternal satisfaction of feeding baby at the breast.

Kim Campbell, Internet

(Continued from previous page) aware, however, of its effect on both the mother's and the baby's liver. Other drugs are available such as Sporonax, but little is known about how they affect the nursing relationship, so mothers might want to ask for another alternative. If a mother chooses to use a prescribed pharmaceutical whose effects are unknown (check with the Professional Liaison Department of your local La Leche League), remember to let her know that she may be able to pump and dump instead of permanently weaning; however, most pharmaceuticals in this class do not require weaning.

All told, managing yeast can be an exasperating experience for mothers, lay support persons and practitioners. The research on yeast, and in particular breast yeast, has not been disseminated throughout the medical community. One way to actively help this dissemination is to suggest to practitioners that they order both the full-color yeast addendum page and the Lactation Series No. 18 Candidiasis and Lactation, available from La Leche League International.

Editor's note: *These treatments are only suggestions. Please consult a naturopathic and/or allopathic practitioner to help you choose a treatment that will be most beneficial and least harmful to mother and baby.*

References:
Hancock, Spangler. (1993). There's a fungus among us! *J Human Lactation* 9(3).
Hansen, R. C., et al. (1993). Candida breast lesions associated with cases of persistent sore nipples: Collaboration between lactation consultant and dermatologist. *J Human Lactation* 9(3): 155-60.
John, C. L., and Cherry, J. D. (1964). Congenital cutaneous candidiasis. *Pediatrics* 33: 440-441.
Kaufmann, R., and Fosman, B. (1991). Mastitis among lactating women. *Soc Sci and Med* 33:701.
Lau, B. (1991). *Garlic Research Update.* Vancouver, B.C.: Odyssey Publishing.
Lawrence, R. A. (1994). *Breastfeeding: A Guide for the Medical Profession.* 4th ed. Philadelphia, Pa.: Mosby Co., pp. 264-265, 492-494.
Lesher, J., Levine, N., and Treadwell, R. (1994, Jan. 30). Fungal skin infections: Common but stubborn. *Patient Care,* pp. 16-44.
Lucas, R. M. (1991). *Miracle Medicinal Herbs.* New York: Parker Publishing, p. 16.
Murray, M., and Pizzorno, J. (1991). *Encyclopedia of Natural Medicine.* Rocklyn, Calif.: Prima Publishing, pp. 186-188.
Newman, J. (1996). When breastfeeding is not contraindicated. Paper presented at the 1996 U.S. Western Division La Leche League Conference in Anaheim, Calif., July 30 to Aug. 4, 1996.
Ogle, K. S., and Davis, S. (1998). Mastitis in lactating women. *J Family Practice* 26(2): 139-144.
Olsen, G., and Gordon, R. (1990). Breast disorders in nursing mothers. *Am Fam Phys* 45(5): 1509-16.
Pessi, M. (1996). Mastitis and yeast. Presentation of the 1996 La Leche League of Oregon Area Conference "To Love a Child," Shilo Inn Suites: Portland, Ore.
Prentice, A. (1985). Mastitis in rural Gambian mothers and protection of the breast by milk antimicrobial factors. *Trans Royal Soc Tropical Hyg,* pp. 79-90.
Riordan, J., and Auerback, K.G. (1993). Candidiasis/thrush, in Riordan and Auerbach, eds., *Breastfeeding and Human Lactation.* Boston: Jones and Bartlett.
Rosa, C., et al. (1990). Yeasts from human milk collected in Rio de Janeiro, Brazil. *Rev Microbiology* 21(4): 361.
Tadi, P. P., Teel, R. W., and Lau, B. H. S. (1990). Anticandidal and anticarcinogenic potentials of garlic. *Intern Clin Nutr Rev* 10: 423-429.
Thomsen, A. D. (1985). Course and treatment of milk stasis, non-infectious inflammation of the breast, and infectious mastitis in nursing women. *Am J Obstet/Gynecol* 149: 492-5.
Trowbridge, J. R., and Walker, M. (1986). *The Yeast Syndrome.* New York: Bantam Books.
Truss, C. O. (1981). The toll of candida albicans in human illness. *J Orthomolecular Psychiatry* 10:228.
Truss, C. O. (1986). *The Missing Diagnosis.* Birmingham, Ala.: Missing Diagnosis, Inc.
Weed, Susun. (1986). *The Wise Woman Herbal for the Childbearing Years.* Woodstock, N.Y.: Ash Tree Publishing, p. 109.

Tips & Tricks

A Bit of Saliva

Thrush does not occur in the healthy adult mouth, but it can seem impossible to get rid of in a baby's mouth. I have seen rapid and marvelous results from having the mom put a bit of her saliva in her baby's mouth after feedings. This is often an effective remedy for even the most resistant cases.

Natalya Lukin, CA

Oil of Oregano

My favorite remedy for thrush/yeast infections is oil of oregano! It has been performing very well on fungal, viral and bacterial infections.

Being a lactation consultant I mostly deal with breastfeeding problems, and the number of yeast infections is just tremendous these days. Sore nipples from yeast have been responding almost immediately and some had already been through the Nystatin route without relief. Most use two drops under the tongue three times a day (it is really strong so a water chaser is helpful, or it can be put in juice). Two drops in a teaspoon of olive oil and rubbed on baby's feet can treat them. That same solution can be applied topically to the nipple.

When I have used it my husband tells me I have the breath of a thousand pizzas!

PJ Jacobsen IBCLC (E-News)

Ice Is Nice

A newly breastfeeding mom who may have painful nipples can rub them with ice. It feels good, and it keeps the baby from latching on too vigorously. The baby will begin to suck slowly, giving the mom a chance to adjust.

Faith Heise, FL

Increasing Milk Supply

To increase milk when mine gets low, I have found that Mother's Milk tea, made by Traditional Medicinals, works well. If I drink one cup in the morning and another cup around noon, I am nearly dripping by afternoon. Even one cup in a day makes a significant difference. It contains fennel seed, anise seed, coriander seed, spearmint leaf, lemongrass, lemon verbena leaf, althea root, blessed thistle leaf and fenugreek seed, a good-tasting combination. This tea is available at some health food stores and is also available from Cascade Healthcare Products or Blooming Prairie Co-op.

The other "herbal" remedy (broadly speaking) I have found effective for increasing milk is oats. When my milk has gotten low, I eat a generous serving of oatmeal for breakfast. Later in the day I can see a difference in the quantity of my milk. I continue to eat this for a few days until my milk is re-established at a sufficient level.

Of course, these remedies should be combined with the common sense solutions of plenty of liquids for mom and enough rest. Making milk is hard work for a mom's body.

K. (E-News)

Midwifery Today, Inc., publications

Midwifery Today magazine
- The only professional midwifery quarterly magazine intended for all midwives, of any definition, worldwide.
- An essential birth resource for midwives, doulas, nurses, childbirth educators and other birth practitioners.
- A great mix of technical, political and narrative articles.
- 72 packed pages every quarter.

Midwifery Today
2 years: —U.S. $95 —Mex/Can $113 —All other Int'l $143
1 year: —U.S. $50 —Mex/Can $60 —All other Int'l $75

The Birthkit
2 years: —U.S. $35 —Mex/Can $41 —All other Int'l $45
1 year: —U.S. $20 —Mex/Can $23 —All other Int'l $25

Having a Baby Today
2 years: —U.S. $35 —Mex/Can $41 —All other Int'l $45
1 year: —U.S. $20 —Mex/Can $23 —All other Int'l $25

The Birthkit newsletter
- Ad-free
- 12-page newsletter
- Birth stories, research, techniques, remedies

Our readers asked us if we could publish *Midwifery Today* magazine more often than quarterly. We couldn't, but we did start *The Birthkit* as an in-between issue fix for those people who just couldn't wait three months for their next issue of *Midwifery Today* to come out.

Save with Special One-year Combo Subscription Rates:
Midwifery Today & *The Birthkit* for one year each, $67
Midwifery Today & *Having a Baby Today* for one year each, $67
Having a Baby Today & *The Birthkit* for one year each, $37
All three publications for one year each, $84

Having a Baby Today newsletter for parents
Having a Baby Today is more specific to the childbearing year than many other alternative publications, and it specifically addresses issues from nutrition to interventions in ways that will enhance existing client education packets and reinforce the messages families need to hear about healthy birth. Call us at 1-800-743-0974 to ask about our great bulk rates!

Great Resources at www.midwiferytoday.com

Secure online shopping cart
Buy books, videos—indeed, anything we sell on the Web—24 hours a day.
Just click on the shopping cart icon.

E-News
Receive free birth information in your e-mail box each week. With more than 10,800 subscribers (as of September 2001) sharing their insight and experience, this FREE newsletter is a terrific resource for anyone interested in birth!
www.midwiferytoday.com/enews

Forums
Riveting reads for your birthing needs! Need a few quick answers from experienced midwives, doulas and moms? Want to share your favorite "Trick of the Trade"?
Visit Midwifery Today's free forums:
www.midwiferytoday.com/forums

Birth Market product and services directory
Find great products or find a midwife, doula or childbirth educator. Shop, recommend or include your practice. Browse through more than 235 birth-related listings!
www.birthmarket.com

www.havingababytoday.com
Midwifery Today's sister site for parents has great resources for parents on waterbirth, homebirth, breastfeeding and much more. Havingababytoday.com makes a perfect starting point for parents on the Web.

Up-to-date conference information
Registration forms, hotel recommendations and programs. Plan for your next CEUs or midwifery intensives!

Midwifery Today, Inc.
P.O. Box 2672 • Eugene, OR USA 97402
800-743-0974 or 541-344-7438
Fax: 541-344-1422
E-mail: inquiries@midwiferytoday.com
www.midwiferytoday.com

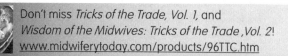
Don't miss *Tricks of the Trade, Vol. 1,* and *Wisdom of the Midwives: Tricks of the Trade, Vol. 2*!
www.midwiferytoday.com/products/96TTC.htm